Meals for Two
Low Carb Recipe Magic

Rene Averett

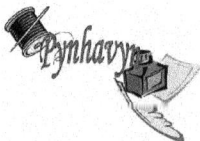

ISBN-13: 978-1942622000 (Pynhavyn Press)
ISBN-10: 1942622007

DEDICATION

This book is dedicated to my grandmother, Lillian Tatum Wulfjen, who was my first teacher in the kitchen. She would be amazed at how far the little girl who created the brick biscuits has come. And it's dedicated to my grandfather, Albert F. Wulfjen, who determinedly ate those brick biscuits. I thank you both and I miss you.

Contents

Introduction 9

Appetizers 12

    Asparagus Bacon Roll Ups..13
    Bacon Cheese Bites 14
    Cauliflower Cheese Puffs...15
    Crab Rangoon Dip 16
    Cranberry Apple Quesadillas 17
    Cranberry & Chicken Wedges 18
    Cranberry & Pear Tarts...21
    E-Z Turkey or Ham Roll Ups...22
    Stuffed Mini-Peppers 23
    Chorizo Sausage Appetizers 24
    Sun-Dried Tomato Spinach Puffs......................................25
    Turkey Tamale Stuffed 'Shrooms 26

Breakfast 27

    Bacon & Avocado Omelet..28
    Breakfast Pizza 29
    Welsh Egg Melts 30
    Cheddar Cornmeal Pancakes 31
    Cream Cheese Waffles 32
    Cream Scone with Quince Apple Preserves.......................33
    Coconut Flour & Almond Flour Cream Scones 34
    Huevos Rancheros de Primavera 35
    Irish Blueberry Fritters 38
    Lasagna Baked Eggs 39
    Mexicali Baked Eggs 40
    Peachy Pecan Pancakes 41
    Scottish Eggs...42
    Turnip & Sausage Frittata 43
    Quick Bake French Toast 44

Brunch 45

    Asian Fusion Dirty Cauli-Rice...46
    Asparagus & White Cheese Quiche 47
    Bacon, Tomato & Broccoli Pie 48
    Chicken à la King 49
    Chicken Tacos with Cucumber Salsa 50
    Deviled Ham Strata 51
    Chicken & Mushroom Crepes 54
    Egg Foo Yung 55
    Mexican Personal Pizza 56
    Sierra Tuna Melt..57
    Pollo Pequitos (Little Chickens) 58
    Sausage Zucchini Bake..59

Shrimp & Asparagus with Cheese Grits 60
Walnut Chicken Salad 61

Dynamic Dinners 62

Artichoke & Peppers Chicken Casserole...............................63
Braised Short Ribs..64
Butternut Squash & Chicken Tostado......................................65
Chicken Cordon Bleu..66
Chicken Provolone Blanca 69
Rene's Coconut Shrimp 70
Cranberry Mustard Baked Salmon...71
Italian Meatloaf for Two 72
Lasagna Carbonara 73
Rene's Pasta Sauce From Scratch 74
Orange Chicken with Bean Sprouts 75
Parmesan Crusted Chicken 76
Chicken Angelica..77
Peanut Curried White Fish 78
Pecan Crusted Chicken..79
Pork, Butternut & Apple Sauté'..80
Pumpkin Shrimp Curry 81
Salmon Cakes With Dill Sauce...82
Creamy Dill Sauce 83
Feline Version...83
Irish Style Salmon With Bacon and Cabbage.........................86
Salsa Chicken...87
Crab Stuffed Cod 88
Quick Poached White Fish 89
Scalloped Chicken & Turnips..90
Simple Salisbury Steak..91
Pork Chile Verde...92
Tempura Cod and Vegetables..93
Tempura Batter 94

Super Sides..95

Avocado Cucumber Salad 96
E-Z Vegetable Fries..96
Broccoli Salad 97
Asparagus & Leek Cauli-Risotto...98
Grandma's Tex-Mex Spanish Cauli-rice 99
Green Cauli Rice...100
Home-style Veggies O'Brien 101
Mexicali Esparragus con el Nabo 104
Orange & Pecan Roasted Brussels Sprouts 105
Smashed Turnips with Cauliflower & Cheddar..........................106
Springtime Coleslaw 107
Turnip & Cauliflower Gratin 108
Zucchini, Spinach & Bacon Fritters 109

Devine Desserts 110

    Almond Tea Biscuits 112
    Caramel Nut Cheesecake 113
    Coconut Flour Flaugnarde 114
    Cranberry Pumpkin Biscotti Cookies 115
    Cranberry Peach Cobbler 116
    Espresso Hazelnut Custard & Bourbon Sauce 119
    Blueberry Dumplings 120
    Peanut Butter Blossom Cookies 121
    Peanut Butter Chocolate Cake 122
    Raspberry Lemon Drop Tart 123
    Sour Cream Lemon Cake 124
    Cranberry Chocolate Pecan Pie Tarts 125
    Pumpkin Cheese Mousse 126
    Pumpkin Flan 127
    Chocolate Mist Cheesecake 128

Breads 129

    Baked Low Carb Crumpets 130
    Baked Tortilla Chips 131
    Cream Cheese Biscuit 132
    Peanut Butter Surprise Muffin 133
    Flat Bread Crackers 134
    Flax Meal Muffin or Roll 137
    Irish Soda Bread 138
    Greek Yogurt Muffin 139
    Simple Crepes 140
    Cheese Taco Shells 141
    Flax Meal Focaccia Bread 142

Special Ingredients 143

Conversion Tables 145

Introduction

You might be wondering who I am and why I am writing a low carb cookbook. Well, I am just a regular gal, who has fought with my weight all my life. If there's a diet out there, I have probably tried it. From childhood on, my weight has been an issue... a BIG issue!

I've lost weight, I've regained weight and it always comes back with friends. I have even lost weight using the Atkins Diet twice before and gained that weight back also. So what is different this time?

For the first time, I feel I have an understanding of how my body uses food and I think that is key to losing and maintaining weight loss. I also understand that losing the weight isn't the entire program. It's a lifestyle change. What you do to lose the weight is what you must continue to do to keep the weight off. If that means exercise and restricted eating, then prepare to continue to do it to maintain that weight loss. Sure, you can add some of your favorite foods back, but you cannot go back to the old habits that added the pounds in the first place.

This is a lesson it took me many, many years to learn. I had hit a new high of 315 pounds on my 5 foot 10 inch frame. Way too much weight! And I was in my mid-sixties. It's harder to lose weight as you get older. A painful, month-long bout with kidney stones in February 2010 reduced my weight by about 27 pounds in less than 25 days. I was determined to keep that weight off and try to add to the loss. By the end of the year, I had lost 38 pounds total. Not exactly stellar. I was frustrated and annoyed with myself.

In February 2011, I went back to the Atkins low carb diet and found that it had been revised. I picked up the *New Atkins for a New You* book and read it through. There were so many changes since the last time I had gone on Atkins and this new version was a much more balanced diet than it had been previously. I decided to try it again. And it worked!

Not quickly, especially because my exercise level is very low. I am not one to go running down the street daily or hang out at the gym. Low impact exercise, maybe. Nothing strenuous. But the pounds came off over the next three years. While I am still a little over my ideal weight, and the weight loss is very slow now, I am at least in the healthy range. To be honest, I am OK with getting into my size 10 jeans and feeling great. If the rest of the weight doesn't come off, that is fine with me.

This brings me to this cookbook. Once I came to the realization that this is a lifestyle change, I also realized that in order to succeed, I needed to adapt. By that, I mean recipes! I love food. I love the taste of the various foods from different cultures – Mexican, Italian, Greek, Thai – you name it. It's a joy in life and it is not something I wanted to give up forever. So adapting the recipes to stay within the low carb requirements became my mission.

Why for two? Because there are many people who are like me. Living with another person, but there's just the two of you and you don't want to make recipes for 6 meals and have the leftovers every night until they're gone. Or worse, left in the refrigerator until they go bad or stuck in the freezer and forgotten.

Because there are people who are the only ones in their home trying to eat a low carb diet while the rest of the family chow down on hamburgers and French fries.

Everyone of these recipes can be easily doubled for more people and most of them don't use special ingredients, unless you count sugar substitutes and almond flour, both of which are readily available at most supermarkets.

The whole family can enjoy most of these without realizing that they are also eating low carb, healthful foods. And you don't have to be on a low carb diet, be it Atkins or South Beach or any other version, in order to cook and enjoy them.

My motto is simply, "Eating low carb doesn't have to be boring."

Rene Averett
Reno, Nevada – February 2015

Author's Note

I had hoped to print this book with full color photographs of the foods; however, that is proving to run the cost of the printed book to something that is unreasonable for a book this size. I have changed all the photos to grayscale and even though it doesn't do justice to the food, it does give you an idea of each item. But, I figure that it's better to have a book you can afford than one that is just too pricey.

I am putting the color pages up on my blog site [http://reneaverett.me/skinnygirl/] where you can view them. Also the Kindle copy will have the color images in it.

Appetizers

What better way to start a recipe book than with meal starters? Or just plain snacks if you prefer.

This chapter offers small batches of low carb, satisfying bites to begin a meal, snack on in the afternoon or just make your meal, depending on how hungry you are.

Asparagus Bacon Roll Ups	13
Bacon Cheese Bites	14
Cauliflower Cheese Puffs	15
Crab Rangoon Dip	16
Cranberry Apple Quesadillas	17
Cranberry & Chicken Wedges	18
Cranberry & Pear Tarts	21
E-Z Turkey or Ham Roll Ups	22
Stuffed Mini-Peppers	23
Chorizo Sausage Appetizers	24
Sun-Dried Tomato Spinach Puffs	25
Turkey Tamale Stuffed 'Shrooms	26

Asparagus Bacon Roll Ups

Super easy recipe that was inspired by a recipe from my grocery store with several changes made by me to make it low carb and more flavorful. These are great to take to work for lunch or a snack. You can substitute broccolini for the asparagus. (Pictured on page 19.)

2 low carb Tortillas, 3 net carbs each
2 slices Bacon, cooked till crisp, drained and crumbled
2 ounces Cream Cheese, room temperature
8 Asparagus Spears
1/8 teaspoon Garlic Pepper seasoning
1/8 teaspoon Italian Seasoning
2 tablespoons Soft Cheese, such as Queso Fresco
1/2 dried Sweet Pepper, crushed
1 tablespoon Melted Butter

Bring a pot of water to a boil and put the trimmed asparagus in it for 2 minutes. Remove to a colander to drain, then dry on a paper towel.

Cut each tortilla in half. Combine the bacon, cream cheese, seasonings, peppers and soft cheese and spread an even layer of the mixture on each tortilla half.

Place 2 asparagus spears, one on end of each tortilla slice, and roll up each slice like a jellyroll. Place seam side down on a lightly greased cookie sheet.

Preheat broiler. Brush the tops and sides of the roll-ups with melted butter. Broil 6 inches from the heat until lightly browned and toasted, about 4 minutes.

Serve Immediately. Makes 4 roll ups.

Nutrition Information: (per roll up)
  Calories: 129.6 Fat: 10 g Net Carbs: 3.3 g Protein: 6.7 g

To store, wrap each half in plastic wrap or put them in a sealable plastic bag. Reheat in the microwave for about 30 seconds or eat cold or at room temperature.

Rene Averett

Bacon Cheese Bites

Simple to make. These Bacon Cheese Bites are bursting with favorite flavors. Serve on flax meal crackers or on sliced zucchini spears. Cut the zucchini lengthwise, then cut slice in half. (Pictured on page 19.)

2 slices Bacon, cooked and crumbled
1/4 cup shredded Sharp Cheddar Cheese
1 teaspoon Dijon Mustard
1/4 cup Mayonnaise
1/8 teaspoon Cayenne Pepper
2 tablespoons Scallions, chopped
8 Flax Meal Crackers (recipe on page 134)

Preheat oven to broil. Prepare broiler pan with aluminum foil.

In a medium bowl combine the mustard and mayonnaise and mix well. Stir in bacon and cheese. Arrange crackers or zucchini slices on broiler pan and spoon mixture onto each slice of bread.

Broil for 2 to 3 minutes, or until lightly brown. Makes 8 appetizers.

Nutrition Information Topping Only – per appetizer.
Calories: 71.8 Fat: 7.0 g Net Carbs: 0.2 g Protein: 2.0 g

Cauliflower Cheese Puffs

While these don't really puff up and they aren't crisp, they are very tasty and a bit like a mashed potato plank. (Pictured on page 19.)

1/4 head of Cauliflower (about 1 cup)	3/4 cup Mozzarella Cheese
2 tablespoons Ricotta Cheese	1 Egg
1/2 teaspoon Cayenne Pepper	Salt and Pepper to taste
1 teaspoon Italian Seasonings	1 teaspoon Garlic Powder
2 tablespoons Bacon Bits (optional)	

Preheat oven to 400 degrees (F). Prepare a pan with parchment paper or foil and spray with baking spray.

Cut the cauliflower into small pieces and chop in the blender until it is finely riced. Add the cheese and pulse a few times to mix the cheese in. Add the seasonings and egg, then pulse again to mix. Through the feeder add one tablespoon of ricotta cheese and pulse for about 10 seconds. Add the second tablespoon and run continuously until the mixture resembles mashed potatoes.

Put the mixture into a quart plastic bag, squeeze out most of the air, then cut the bottom tip on one side of the bag to make a narrow funnel. Pipe the batter onto the prepared pan in about one and a half inch long bars. Leave room between each bar as they will puff out some. They don't puff up, but they do expand.

Bake for 20 minutes, then flip the puffs over and bake an additional 10 minutes until they are golden brown.

If you wish to add chopped bacon to the mix, stir it in by hand before filling the piping bag.

Makes about 40 puffs - number will vary so I've included the whole recipe total.

Nutrition Info: Based on 40 puffs
   Calories: 11 Fat: 0.4 g Net Carbs: 0.4 g Protein: 0.9 g

Whole Recipe Nutrition Info:
   Calories: 440 Fat: 24.3 g Net Carbs: 16.1 g Protein: 35.2 g

Crab Rangoon Dip

This is an elegant and rich-tasting hot dip that is easily made. For dippers, you can use Baked Tortilla Chips (see page 131), Pork Rinds or Cauliflower or Broccoli flowerets. You can also make it with lobster instead of crab. (Pictured on page 19.)

1/4 cup Crabmeat
2 oz. Cream Cheese, softened
2 tablespoons Sour Cream
2 tablespoons Green Onion, chopped
2 drops Worcestershire Sauce
Dash Garlic Powder
1/4 teaspoon Cayenne Pepper
2 drops Lemon Juice

Dippers:
2 Low Carb Tortillas or 12 Pork Rinds
  Or Cauliflower or Broccoli flowerets

Preheat oven to 350 degrees (F.)

Set the cream cheese out 30 minutes to an hour before starting to let it soften.

Add chopped green onions to crabmeat. Mix the cream cheese until it is smooth. Add the sour cream, Worcestershire sauce, garlic powder and lemon juice. Stir until mixed together, then stir in the crabmeat.

Butter a small baking dish. Spoon the dip mixture into the dish.

Bake for 25 to 30 minutes until the dip is bubbly. Remove and let sit for 5 minutes, then serve with dippers. Makes 2 servings.

Nutrition Information for Dip 1 serving
  Calories: 157.6 Fat:12.7 g Net Carbs: 2.6 g Protein: 9.0 g

Cranberry Apple Quesadillas

I saw this recipe in a magazine and thought it would be excellent adapted for low carb, which is where most of the changes are in it. I was not wrong. It's a great appetizer or eat as a meal. For those who are the lower phases of Atkins, the apple isn't an approved fruit, but the carbs fall within the range. Maybe for a treat? (Pictured on page 19.) The crepe recipe is on page 140.

2 teaspoons Butter
2 tablespoons Sweet Onion, diced
1/4 Green Apple, peeled and chopped
2 tablespoons fresh Cranberries chopped
1/2 cup Chicken Breast, chopped or shredded
2 low carb Flour Tortillas, 6 inch size or four 4 inch Crepes
1/2 cup shredded Jack Cheese or Cheddar Jack Cheese

Preheat oven to 400 degrees (F.) Spray a baking pan or cookie sheet with cooking spray.

Melt butter in a skillet and add onion, apples and cranberries. Cook for 10 minutes over low heat, stirring frequently. Remove from heat.

Spread 1/2 the mixture over each tortilla, top with 1/2 the chicken on each tortilla, then add 1/2 the cheese to the tortillas. Fold in half and place each folded tortilla on the baking sheet. If using crepes, put ¼ of the filling and chicken on each crepe and fold in half.

Bake for 10 minutes or until the tortillas are crisp and the cheese is melted. Cut into four slices and serve. For crepes, cut each crepe in half.

Makes 8 appetizers or a meal for two people.

Nutrition Information for one appetizer
  Calories: 65.6 Fat: 3.8 g Net Carbs: 1.7 g Protein: 5.8 g

Nutrition Information for one lunch or dinner serving
  Calories: 262.6 Fat: 15.2 g Net Carbs: 6.9 g Protein: 23.4 g

Cranberry & Chicken Wedges

Want a really great snack for game day? This recipe, inspired by one from my local grocery store, is wonderful. Another easy one on a tortilla base, you can make these up ahead of time, cover with plastic wrap and then bake just before serving. (Pictured on page 19.)

2 Low-Carb Tortillas, 6 or 7 inches*
3/4 cup Chicken or Turkey, chopped
1/4 cup Bacon Bits
1 medium Scallion, chopped
3/4 cup Shredded Italian Blend Cheese
2 tablespoons Cranberries, chopped
3 tablespoons Mayonnaise
2 tablespoons Parmesan Cheese, grated
1 tablespoon Heavy Whipping Cream
1/2 teaspoon Italian Seasonings

Preheat oven to 425 degrees F. Spray a baking sheet with cooking spray. Place tortillas on top.

In a small bowl, mix together the mayonnaise, cream and grated Parmesan. Spread half of the mixture on each of the tortillas. Spread half the chopped chicken (or turkey), cheese, cranberries, bacon and chopped scallions (green onions) on each tortilla.

Bake for 8 to 10 minutes or until cheese is lightly toasted. Cut each into 4 wedges.

Nutrition per wedge:
  Calories: 114.9 Fat: 6.6 g Net carbs: 1.8 g Protein: 11.6 g

* Can't find tortillas in your stores? You can make your own using riced cauliflower and mozzarella cheese. Mix equal amount of each in your food processor and press into a parchment paper lined round cake pan. Bake for 5 minutes, let cool, then put your toppings on and Bake as directed above. Or you can use a flax meal crackers made into rounds. See the recipe on page 134.

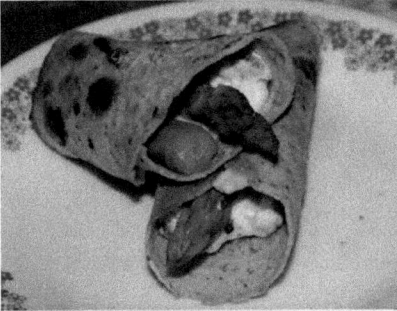

Asparagus Bacon Roll Ups—pg 13

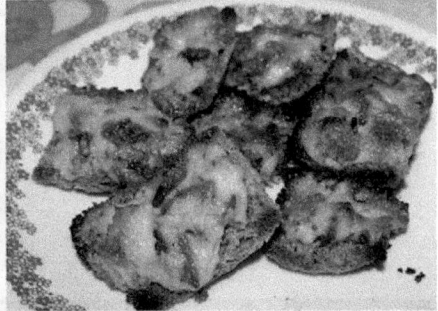

Bacon Cheese Bites—pg 14

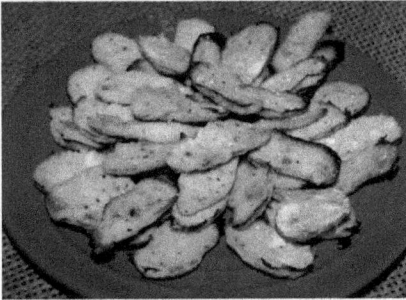

Cauliflower Cheese Puffs—pg 15

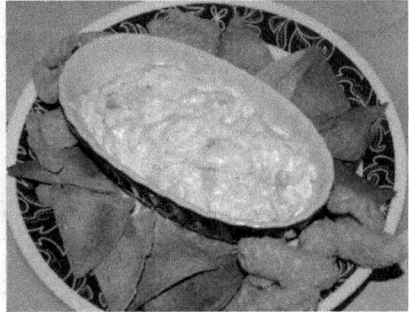

Crab Rangoon Dip—pg 16

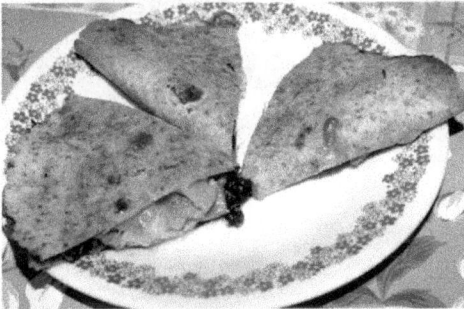

Cranberry Apple Quesadillas—pg 17

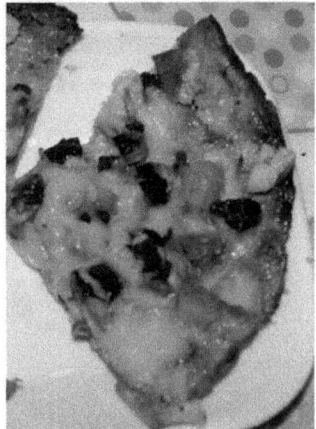

Cranberry & Chicken Wedges—pg 18

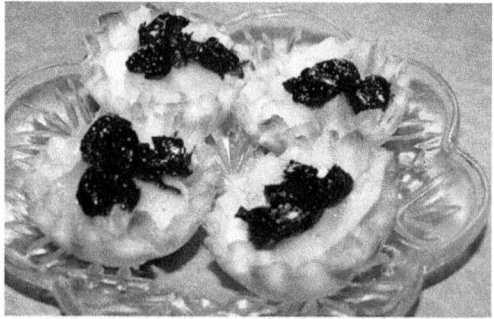

Cranberry & Pear Tarts—pg 21

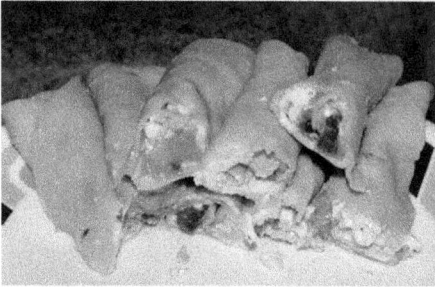

E-Z Turkey Roll Ups—pg 22

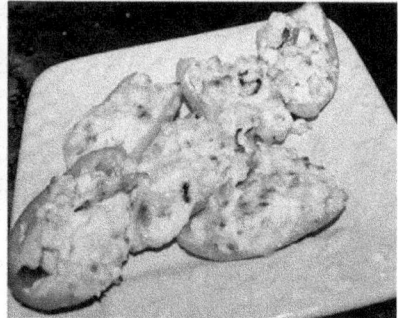

Stuffed Mini-Peppers—pg 23

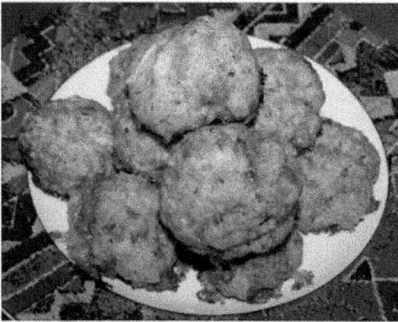

Sausage & Cheese Appetizers—pg 24

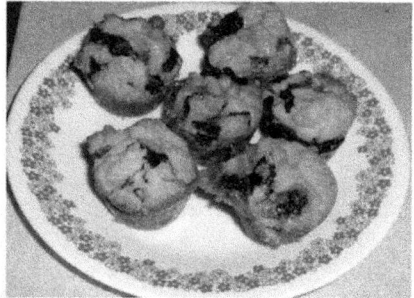

Sun-Dried Tomato Spinach Puffs—pg 25

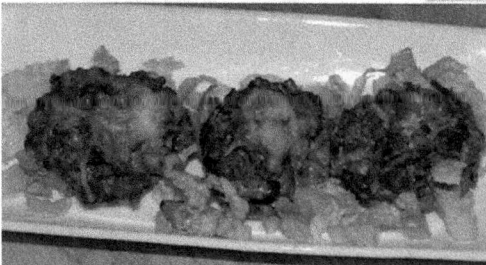

Turkey Tamale Stuffed 'Shrooms—pg 26

Cranberry & Pear Tarts

Cranberries pair wonderfully with pears and Brie cheese in these heavenly-tasting appetizers. Even though these use filo cups, the carb count is pretty low so long as you don't go crazy. These taste so good they could be dessert. (Pictured on page 20.)

8 teaspoons Fresh Pear, chopped
4 teaspoons fresh Cranberries, chopped
1 teaspoon Sugar Substitute
8 teaspoons Brie cheese
8 Athens Filo Dough Mini-Cups

Preheat oven to 350 degrees F. Prepare baking sheet with a piece of parchment paper to cover.

Put filo cups on the parchment paper. Add cinnamon to pears and stir in. I used soft, spreadable Brie cheese, so if you use that, spoon about 1 teaspoon into each cup. If the cheese is harder, slice about the same amount into the cups. Spoon 1 teaspoon of pears on top of the cheese, then spoon 1/2 teaspoon of cranberries on top of that. Using a 1/8 teaspoon measure, sprinkle a little sugar on top of each tart.

Bake for about 12 minutes to just cook the pear and cranberry and meld the cheese flavor into them. Let cool and serve warm or chill and serve cold with a bit of whipped cream for dessert.

Makes 8 tarts, one serving is 2 tarts.

Nutrition Info per tart.
  Calories: 20.6 Fat: 0.9g Net Carbs: 2.8 g Protein: 0.7

E-Z Turkey or Ham Roll Ups

Simple to make for quick party snacks and to take to work. Four of them make a nice lunch with a salad on the side. (Pictured on page 20.)

4 slices of thinly sliced Turkey
1 oz of Cream Cheese
1 teaspoon Heavy Cream or Sour Cream
Mrs. Dash Garlic Pepper seasoning or seasoning of your choice
4 teaspoons of Guacamole or 8 thin slices of Avocado
1 ounce of Queso Fresco or other crumbly cheese

Let cream cheese soften, then mix with heavy cream or sour cream and seasoning until well blended.

Put a slice of turkey on a plate, spread 1/4 of the cream cheese mix onto the slice near the middle. Spread 1 teaspoon of guacamole or place two slices of avocado along the cream cheese. Sprinkle with crumbled queso fresco. Fold one edge of the turkey in and roll it over the filling into a tube. Cut the tube across the middle diagonally. Repeat with the other turkey slices. Makes 8 small appetizers, which is one serving for a solo snack or appetizers for 2.

Nutrition Information per serving:
  Calories: 223.7 Fat: 7.5 g Net Carbs: 4.7 g Protein: 13.2 g

Per each small piece
  Calories: 28   Fat: 2 g   Net Carbs: 0.6 g Protein: 1.7 g

Stuffed Mini-Peppers

Another easy to make party snack that is so yummy and colorful. The little mini-peppers are perfect for stuffing. (Pictured on page 20.)

4 Mini Sweet Peppers (about 1 1/2 inches long)
2 oz Cream Cheese, softened
2 tablespoon Real Bacon Bits
1/4 cup Sharp Cheddar Cheese
1/2 teaspoon Cayenne Pepper
1/4 teaspoon Garlic Powder
1/2 tablespoon Green Onion, chopped

Turn on broiler. Prepare a baking pan that will fit the broiler pan with a sheet of aluminum foil on it. Spray with baking spray.

Cut each pepper in half, remove the stems, seeds and membranes. Dry completely with a paper towel.

Mix cream cheese, onions, cheese and seasonings together until blended. Stuff each pepper with about 1 teaspoon of the filling mix. Put on the baking tray, filling side up.

Put under the broiler for about 5 minutes. Check after four minutes, then check frequently. When lightly browned, remove and serve.

Makes 8 appetizers.

Nutrition Information per appetizer
Calories: 49.8 Fat: 4.0 g Net Carbs: 1.2 g Protein: 2.4 g

Chorizo Sausage Appetizers

Game time or any Sunday afternoon TV viewing is a good time to relax with a few snacks. These little sausage balls are great on their own or when combined with low carb chicken wings, stuffed mini peppers or meat and cheese roll ups. This version uses chorizo sausage, preferably the Texas style or Mexican style that is not as solid as the Basque style. It usually has a chili mixed into the sausage. If you can't find it, use bulk sausage with seasonings. (Pictured on page 20.)

    1/2 cup Chorizo Sausage, Mexican or Texas style
     Or 1/2 cup bulk Sausage with seasonings
    1/4 cup Almond Flour
    2 tablespoon Golden Flax Meal
    1 Egg
    2 tablespoons Ricotta Cheese
    1 tablespoon Heavy Cream
    1/2 cup Cheddar Cheese
    2 tablespoon minced Onions
    1/4 teaspoon Garlic Powder
    1/4 teaspoon Cayenne Pepper
    1 tablespoon, Parsley, chopped

Preheat oven to 350 degrees F. Place a sheet of foil or a silicone mat on a cookie pan and place a cookie rack on top. Spray with cooking spray.

Mix all the ingredients together in a bowl until completely combined. Roll about 1 1/2 tablespoons of mixture into a ball about 1 1/2 inches in diameter. Place on the rack and repeat with the rest of the mixture. It will make 8 large sausage balls.

Bake for 25 to 30 minutes until the meatballs are browned. Allow to cool 5 to 10 minutes to firm up before serving.

Makes 8 sausage balls. Two make a nice-sized appetizer.

Nutrition Info per sausage ball:
  Calories: 142 Fat: 11.7 g Net Carbs: 1.1 g Protein: 7.5 g

Sun-Dried Tomato Spinach Puffs

One of the first recipes I adapted, the original version came from my grocery store. The adjusted version is low carb and considerably different from the original inspiration, but tastes fantastic. (Pictured on page 20.)

Spinach Topping:
1/2 cup Spinach, fresh, chopped & packed
2 tablespoons Scallions, chopped
2 tablespoons Sun Dried Tomatoes, minced
1/4 cup Cheddar Cheese, finely shredded
2 tablespoons Bacon Bits
½ teaspoon Olive Oil

Ricotta Puff Dough
2 large Eggs at room temperature
1/8 teaspoon Cream of Tartar
1 oz Ricotta Cheese
1 tablespoons Low Carb Flour (optional)
1/8 teaspoon Garlic and Herb seasoning

Preheat oven to 300 degrees F.
Using cooking spray, grease a 12 slot mini-muffin pan or insert mini-muffin cups.

Sauté spinach and scallions (or green onions) in olive oil over medium heat for a minute or two until spinach is limp. Stir in minced tomatoes and bacon bits. Set aside.

In a clean bowl, beat egg whites until foamy. Add cream of tartar and beat until stiff.

In another bowl, mix together egg yolks, ricotta cheese and flour. Fold mixture into the egg whites being careful to not beat them down.

Spoon the batter evenly into the muffin cups to about 2/3 full. Bake for five minutes until the batter is just set. Pull out and spoon spinach topping on each puff. Sprinkle shredded cheese on top of the spinach. Return to oven and bake another 10 minutes. Cheese should be melted and lightly toasted.

Makes 12 appetizers

Nutrition Information per appetizer
  Calories: 34 Fat: 2.4 g Net Carbs: 0.5 g Protein: 2.6 g

Turkey Tamale Stuffed 'Shrooms

I am a big fan of stuffed mushrooms. My friends and I used to have frequent stuffed mushroom parties with everyone bringing a favorite mushroom recipe. This is one I concocted for a recent family party. It brings the flavor of a tamale to the mushroom. (Pictured on page 20.)

4 oz. Lean Ground Turkey
1 Egg
2 tablespoons Onions, chopped
2 tablespoons diced green chiles
1 teaspoon Red Chile Powder
1/2 cup Diced Tomatoes
1 tablespoon Black Olives, chopped
2 tablespoons Baby Corn, chopped
1/8 teaspoon Cumin
1/4 cup Shredded Mexican Four Cheese blend
1/4 cup Ricotta Cheese
1 tablespoons Corn Meal or Golden Flax Meal
6-8 large Mushrooms, stems removed and trimmed

Clean mushrooms, remove stems and chop up any useable parts. Dry mushrooms with a paper towel and set on a rack.

Preheat oven to 365 degrees (F.) Spray a baking dish with baking spray or butter.

Mix all the ingredients, including any chopped mushroom stems, together, combining thoroughly.

Use a spoon to stuff each mushroom to completely filled and place in the baking pan.

Cook for 25 to 30 minutes until the sausage is completely cooked and the tops are lightly browned. Serve hot or warm.

Makes 6 to 8 appetizers

Nutrition Information based on 6 appetizers
Calories: 64 Fat: 2.9 g Net Carbs: 1.4 g Protein: 7.1 g

Breakfast

It's the most important meal of the day, or so experts tell us. From a low carb standpoint, it really is good to have a satisfying breakfast that gives your body both protein and some fats. Luckily, there are many ways to fulfill these requirements. Here are some day-starters that are tasty and easy.

Bacon & Avocado Omelet   28
Breakfast Pizza   29
Welsh Egg Melts   30
Cheddar Cornmeal Pancakes   31
Cream Cheese Waffles   32
Cream Scone with Quince Apple Preserves   33
Coconut Flour & Almond Flour Cream Scones   34
Huevos Rancheros de Primavera   35
Irish Blueberry Fritters   38
Lasagna Baked Eggs   39
Mexicali Baked Eggs   40
Peachy Pecan Pancakes   41
Scottish Eggs   42
Turnip & Sausage Frittata   43
Quick Bake French Toast   44

Bacon & Avocado Omelet

Eggs are an almost perfect foods for anyone. They are loaded with nutrition, take a long time to digest and are very low carb. For all of its rich flavor, avocado is surprisingly low carb and is like a reward when you're trying to keep the carbs down. Add in some bacon and salsa and you have a satisfying, tasty breakfast. It also reheats pretty well if you don't put the avocado on until you are ready to eat it. (Pictured on page 36.)

> 3 or 4 large Eggs
> 1/2 Haas Avocado, cut into slices
> 1/4 cup Cheddar Cheese
> 4 tablespoons Southwest Style Salsa (optional)
> 4 slices thick Bacon, crumbled
> Dash Pepper
> 1/4 teaspoon Seasoning Salt
> 1 tablespoon Butter
> 1 tablespoon Water

Break eggs into a bowl, add water, seasoning salt and pepper. Beat or whisk until foamy. Heat a medium-size round bottom pan or omelet pan with 1 tablespoon butter over medium heat.

Add eggs and let cook for a couple of minutes until the egg sets on the bottom, then begin lifting the edges with the spatula and tilting the pan so that the uncooked egg runs underneath. Repeat, working your way around the pan. Keep lifting and tilting until most of the liquid egg is gone. This builds a fluffier omelet.

Evenly distribute the bacon and most of the cheese down one-half of the omelet. Use the spatula to lift and fold the omelet over the top. Reduce heat to low and put a lid over the pan. Let cook for about 3 minutes in order to melt the cheese.

Sprinkle 1 tablespoon of cheese over the top. Cut the omelet in half and serve each half with 2 tablespoons of salsa and half the avocado slices. If you wish, you can heat the salsa before serving.

Makes 2 servings

Nutrition Information per servings
Calories: 430 Fat: 35.3 g Net Carbs: 3.0 g Protein: 23.5 g

Breakfast Pizza

This is a quick, low carb solution to the desire for pizza. It can be a great little breakfast pizza with an egg on top or leave off the egg, add more toppings and make it a lunch pizza. It uses a low carb tortilla for the base. If you can't find them at your supermarket, you can order them from Netrition.com or you can make a cauliflower base version (see page 18). (Pictured on page 36.)

2 Low Carb Tortillas
1 Italian Sausage
4 tablespoons Pasta Sauce
    (look for low carbs - mine is 4 net carbs for 1/2 cup)
1 tablespoon Onion, chopped
2 tablespoons Tomatoes, diced
2 tablespoons Bell Pepper, diced
1/4 cup Mozzarella Cheese
2 tablespoons Parmesan Cheese, shredded
2 eggs (optional)
1/2 teaspoon crushed Red Peppers (optional)

Preheat oven or toaster oven to 350 degrees (F.)

Put tortilla on a baking pan and bake for 5 minutes until the tortilla is lightly browned.

Meanwhile, remove the sausage from the casing and brown in a skillet, breaking it into small pieces. When the tortillas are done, spread ½ the pasta sauce on each tortilla. Add 1/2 of the sausage, spread evenly on top of the sauce. Mix the onions, tomatoes, bell peppers and crushed red peppers, if you are using it, together and distribute 1/2 of the mixture onto each tortilla. Top with 1/2 of the mozzarella cheese and parmesan cheese.

Bake for about 5 to 7 minutes until the cheese is melted and the tortilla is just toasted.

While the pizza bakes, prepare the eggs. I used fried eggs, but you can make them however you prefer or leave them off. Top each pizza with an egg, season and serve.

Makes 2 servings

Nutrition Information per serving:
    Calories:358 Fat: 24.5 g Net Carbs: 6.1 g Protein: 24.9 g

Welsh Egg Melts

Ideally, this recipe should use Welsh White Cheddar cheese or even an Irish White Cheddar, but any good sharp cheddar will work well. It makes a scrumptious breakfast. See the recipe for Flax Meal Focaccia Bread on page 142 or substitute any low carb bread you prefer. (Pictured on page 36.)

4 strips thick-cut Bacon or 2 slices Irish Style Bacon
1 slice low carb Flax Focaccia Bread, cut through the middle
1/2 ripe Avocado, mashed
1/2 cup shredded Welsh (or Irish) White Cheddar Cheese
2 Eggs

In a large skillet, cook the bacon until it is crisp. Drain on paper towels. Lightly toast the bread in the oven or toaster oven. Spread avocado on each slice and top with tomato and bacon. Sprinkle with oregano, then sprinkle cheese on top.

Prepare eggs while the broiler heats. Use either fried or poached eggs on top or scramble your eggs, if you prefer. Salt and pepper to taste.

Place sandwiches on broiler pan or in a pie tin and broil for 2 minutes until the cheese is melted. Top each sandwich with an egg and serve.

Serves two.

Nutrition Info: (with focaccia bread)
  Calories: 327 Fat: 14.8 g Net Carbs: 3.5 g Protein: 18.6 g

Nutrition Info: (without bread)
  Calories: 217 Fat: 17.8 g Net Carbs: 2.4 g Protein: 13.8 g

Cheddar Cornmeal Pancakes

I adapted this recipe for low carb, loosely based on one from the grocery store. It has enough cornmeal to give it flavor without running up the carbohydrates too much. (Pictured on page 36.)

1/4 cup low carb Baking Mix	2 tablespoons Heavy Cream
1 tablespoon Water	1 tablespoon Cornmeal
1 tablespoon Golden Flax Meal	1 Egg, beaten
2 tablespoons Sharp Cheddar, grated	Butter for skillet
1/4 teaspoon Mexican Blend Seasoning	2 fried Eggs
2 tablespoons Fresh Pico de Gallo	2 teaspoons Sour Cream
1/4 cup Ground Beef	1 teaspoon Water
1/4 teaspoon Taco Seasoning	

Heat skillet, break ground beef into pieces and use a spatula to break it smaller for a taco consistency as you stir fry it. Add the taco seasoning and water and mix it into the ground beef. Once the beef is done, turn off the pan, cover and set aside while you make the pancakes.

For the pancakes, stir together baking mix or pancake mix, cream, cornmeal, cheese, seasoning and beaten egg in a medium bowl.

Heat a skillet with butter to coat the bottom over medium heat. Add 1/2 the pancake batter. Cook over medium to low heat until bubbles form and the batter begins to dry out on the top. I like to put a lid over the skillet to speed the cooking process, which reduces the possibility of burning the bottom. Flip after about four minutes and cook the other side 3 to 4 minutes. Repeat for second pancake.

Prepare fried or poached eggs. Assemble with a pancake on the bottom, 1/2 the taco meat on top of the pancake, the egg on the taco meat, then the Pico de Gallo or salsa and sour cream on top.

Nutrition Information per serving
Calories: 481 Fat: 39.1 g Net Carbs: 5.8 g Protein: 23.2 g

Cream Cheese Waffles

Simply the best low carb waffle I've tasted. (Pictured on page 36.) For two whole waffles:

2 large Eggs, separated	2 oz. Cream Cheese
1/4 teaspoon Cream of Tartar	1 teaspoon Baking Powder
1/4 cup Low Carb Baking Mix or Almond Flour	1/2 teaspoon Vanilla Extract
1 tablespoons Vanilla Whey Powder	1 teaspoon Sugar Substitute
	1 tablespoon Coconut Flour

Heat the waffle iron and spray with no stick cooking spray.

In a medium bowl, beat egg whites and cream of tartar until stiff. In another bowl, beat egg yolks and cream cheese until smooth. Add baking powder, flours and whey powder and sugar substitute and mix together.

Fold the egg yolk mixture into the egg whites. Add about 1 tablespoon of water if the mixture is too thick to fold easily into the egg whites. Do not stir or beat the whites as that will break down the air in the whites.

Spoon ½ the mixture into the waffle iron, spreading it around gently. It's easiest to mound a tablespoon full in each section of the waffle iron, then spread it a bit. Close the waffle iron and cook for 2 ½ to 3 minutes. Watch for the steam to quit rising off the waffle iron. Open the lid carefully. If it is done, the lid will lift easily and the waffle won't stick to it. If there is resistance, let it cook a little longer. The waffle should be a golden brown.

Re-spray the iron with cooking spray and repeat with the rest of the batter.

Serve topped with butter and zero carb maple syrup or top with fresh strawberries and whipped cream.

Nutrition Information for 1 waffle, no toppings:
Calories: 270 Fat:7.2 g Net Carbs: 6.5 g Protein: 16.4 g

Cream Scone with Quince Apple Preserves

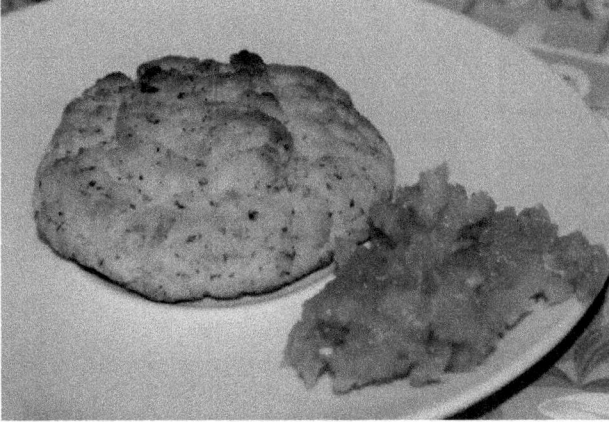

Quince is in season in the fall, so it's the only time to buy these apple-like fruits. I mixed mine with apple although you can make it with just the quince or just the apple. This recipe makes about 1 cup of preserves. If you can't use all that in a couple of weeks, then put half in a freezer bag, remove as much air as possible and freeze for later.

1 Quince	1 Cooking Apple
1 cup Sugar Substitute	1 tablespoon Pectin
2 cups of Water	1 Tablespoon Lemon Juice

Peel and grate, or finely chop, the apple and the quince.

Bring the water to a boil and add the grated or chopped fruit. Let them cook, stirring now and then, until they are soft, about 10 minutes. Add the sugar substitute and lemon juice, lower the cook temperature to medium and continue to cook until the sauce thickens to a jam. Let cool, then ladle into a clean jar and store in refrigerator.

Nutrition Info per tablespoon: (16 servings per recipe)
Calories: 9.7 Fat: 0.0 g Net Carbs: 2.2 g Protein: 0.1 g

Rene Averett

Coconut Flour & Almond Flour Cream Scones

Scones are an easy to make quick bread that are perfect for breakfast or tea time. This recipe uses almond flour and coconut flour. Just be sure to let the scones cool before cutting or moving as these flours have a tendency to break when they are still hot. The extra egg white is needed to give more rise to the scones.

½ cup Almond Flour
¼ cup Sugar Substitute
1 teaspoon Baking Soda
2 tbsp Butter or Shortening
1 Egg White (can use liquid whites)
2 tablespoons Heavy Cream

2 tablespoons Coconut Flour
1 teaspoon Baking Powder
1/4 teaspoon Salt
1 Egg
1 teaspoon Vanilla

Water as needed to produce a stiff, but moist dough.

Preheat oven to 375 degrees (F) and place the rack in the middle of the oven. Line a cookie sheet with parchment paper.

In a large bowl, whisk together the flours, sugar substitute, baking powder, baking soda and salt. Cut the butter into small pieces and use a pastry blender or two knives or your fingers to cut into the mixture until it resembles coarse crumbs. Mix together egg, egg white, vanilla and heavy cream. Add to the flour mixture and stir until just combined. Do not over mix. If dough is too dry, add water a teaspoon at a time. Coconut flour absorbs liquid so the dough may require a few teaspoons to get a biscuit-like consistency.

Knead dough gently four or five times then pat it into a circle that is about 7 inches (18 cm) round. Using a 2 ½ inch cookie cutter or the top of a glass, cut the dough into rounds. Or you can score the top into quarters to make triangular pieces. Brush the tops of the scones with a little cream. This helps to brown the tops of the scones during baking. Let scones rest about 10 minutes before baking.

Bake for about 15 - 18 minutes until nicely browned and a toothpick inserted into the center of a scone comes out clean. Remove from oven and transfer to a wire rack to cool.

Serve with Quince Apple Preserves or any other low carb jam or jelly, butter or clotted cream.

Nutrition Information per scone:
Calories: 189.3 Fat: 17.1 g Net Carbs: 2.5 g Protein: 6.2 g

Huevos Rancheros de Primavera

I call these "spring" ranch eggs because they are best made when asparagus is arriving in supermarkets (or your garden) in the spring. You definitely want to use fresh asparagus for it. If asparagus isn't available, try broccolini (baby broccoli) with it. (Pictured on page 36.)

2 Low Carb Tortillas
2 to 4 Eggs
1/2 link Mexican-style Chorizo or 1/2 cup ground Beef or Pork
1 – 2 oz. Queso Blanco or Queso Fresco cheese
1/2 cup Enchilada Sauce (canned or homemade)
3 tablespoons Pico de Gallo
2 tablespoons Chipotle Salsa or other Salsa
6 spears of Asparagus or Broccolini
2 tablespoons Sour Cream

Preheat oven to 365 degrees F.

Wash and trim the asparagus spears. Bring a pot of water to a boil and put the asparagus spears in for two minutes to blanch. Remove and drain the spears.

Prepare a baking sheet with cooking spray or parchment paper to prevent sticking. Put enchilada sauce in a pie pan and dip each tortilla in it, making sure the whole tortilla is covered. Place on the baking sheet and put in the hot oven for 10 minutes.

Remove the chorizo from its casing and stir fry it in a small skillet until it is done. In another skillet, fry the eggs the way you like them. Or poach the eggs. Or you can scramble the eggs with the chorizo. Mix the salsa with the Pico de Gallo in a small bowl.

Put a tortilla on the plate, arrange 3 asparagus spears in a trio with the bottoms meeting and the tops spread across the tortilla. Put the egg on top, then put the chorizo around the edge of the eggs. Put a little salsa on each side and across the tops of the spears. Crumble queso fresco or Queso Blanco over the entire tortilla, about 2 to 3 tablespoons, then put sour cream on top of the egg. Add salt and pepper, if desired and serve immediately.
Serves 2.

Nutrition Information:
Calories: 263.7 g Fat: 18.1 g Net Carbs: 8.4 g Protein: 14.4 g

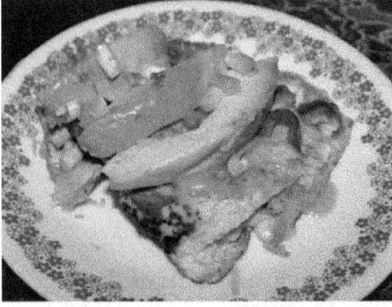
Avocado Bacon Omelet—pg 28

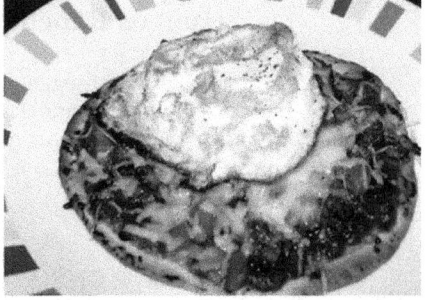
Breakfast Pizza—pg 29

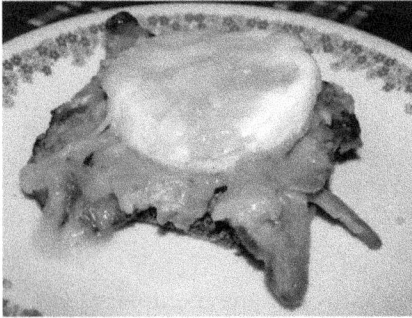
Welsh Cheddar Melt—pg 30

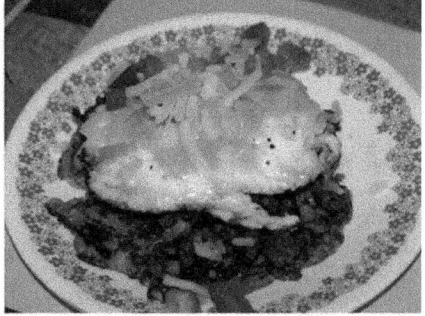
Cheddar Cornmeal Pancakes—pg 31

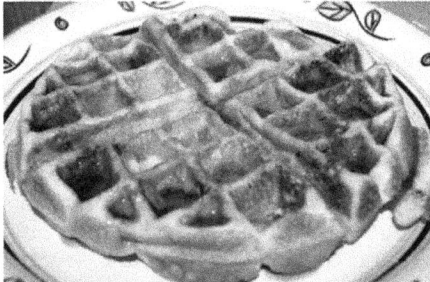
Cream Cheese Waffles—pg 32

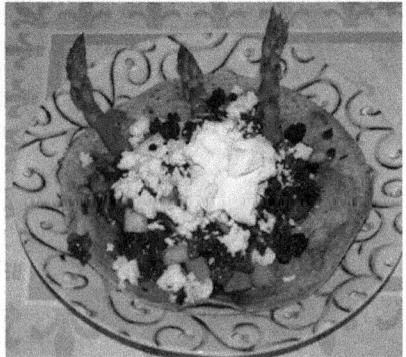
Huevos Rancheros de Primavera—pg 35

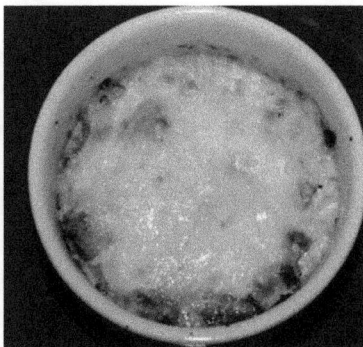

Lasagna Baked Eggs—pg 39

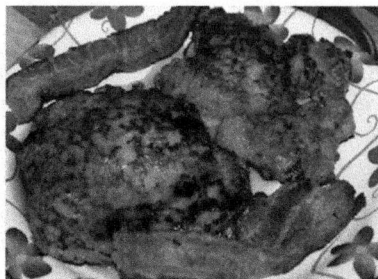

Irish Blueberry Fritters—pg 38

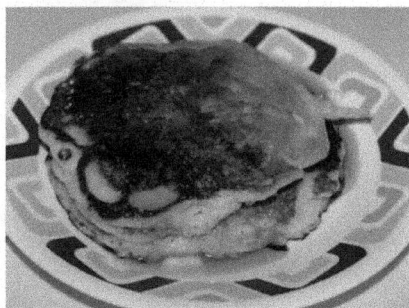

Mexicali Baked Egg—pg 40

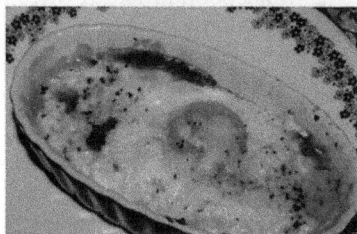

Peachy Pecan Pancakes—pg 41

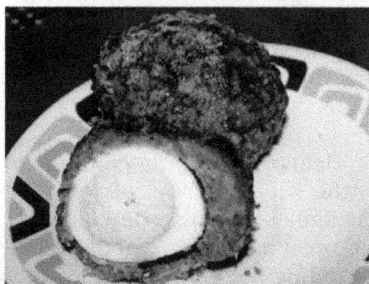

Scottish Eggs—pg 42

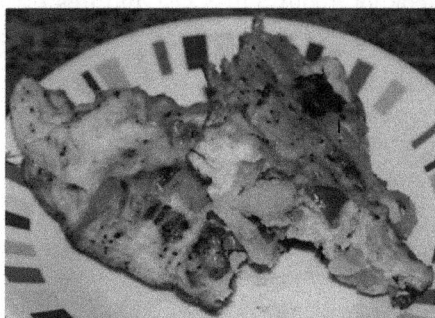

Turnip & Sausage Frittata—pg 43

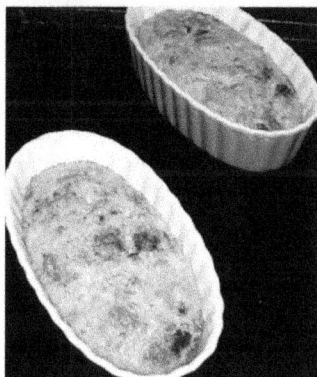

Quick Bake French
Toast — pg 44

Irish Blueberry Fritters

This is a cross between French toast and a fritter. It's cooked in skillet like French toast from a bread and egg mix rather than a dough, but it resembles a fritter. Soda Bread recipe on pg. 138. (Pictured on page 37.)

Makes two servings

2 wedges Irish Soda Bread (low carb)
1large Egg
1/4 cup Almond Milk
  OR 2 tablespoons each Heavy Cream & Water
2 tablespoons Ricotta Cheese
1 teaspoon Cinnamon
1/4 teaspoon Clove
1 teaspoon Vanilla
1/4 cup fresh or frozen Blueberries, drained
1 tablespoon Sugar Substitute
1 tablespoon Butter
1/4 cup chopped Pecans or Walnuts (optional)

Mix egg, ricotta cheese, cream or milk, water, cinnamon, clove, vanilla and sugar substitute together in a small mixing bowl. Crumble the Irish soda bread into the bowl and add the nuts (if using). Mix well with a tablespoon and let it sit until all the liquid is absorbed. If the mix is too dry, add a tablespoon more of cream and mix it in. It should be a lumpy batter.

Heat a skillet on medium heat and melt the butter into it. When the butter begins to sizzle, spoon 1/4 of the batter (about 2 tablespoons) into the skillet making evenly sized (about 2 ½ to 3 inch) patties. Cover with a domed pan lid or tent with foil. Cook for about 3 to 3 1/2 minutes, adjusting the heat a little lower if they are cooking too quickly. Flip the patties and cook that side another 2 ½ to 3 minutes until it is browned.

Butter the fritters and sprinkle cinnamon sugar over the top or serve with sugar free syrup. A slice of bacon or sausage adds to the meal.

Makes 2 servings

Nutrition Information per serving
  Calories: 386.9 Fat: 15.4 g Net Carbs: 7.1 g Protein: 9.8 g

Lasagna Baked Eggs

Bring a little Italian flavor to breakfast or brunch with these easy to make eggs. You can add a little mozzarella cheese on top. I use one egg in each serving, but if you would like a little more, just add a second egg. It only adds a little to the overall carb count. (Pictured on page 37.)

½ cup Marinara Sauce
½ teaspoon crushed Dried Peppers
4 slices of Zucchini, 1/4 inch thick
2 or 3 sprinkles Italian Herbs
2 tablespoons Reggiano, finely shredded
4 teaspoons Olive Oil
2 tablespoon Ricotta Cheese
2 Eggs
2 Pork Sausage Patties
Salt and Pepper

Preheat oven to 425 degrees F.

In a small oven-proof baking dish or two single-serving casseroles, spray the bottom with cooking spray, then spoon ¼ cup (2 tablespoons if using individual casseroles) of the Marinara sauce on the bottom and top with the sliced zucchini. Spoon the rest of the Marinara sauce on top. Spread the ricotta cheese on top (1 tablespoon in each dish if using 2.)

In a small skillet, cook the sausage, breaking it into small pieces. Use a spoon to make a slight well in the ricotta and arrange the sausage around the well. If using a single dish, space these at least three inches apart.

Break an egg in a recipe bowl or small bowl being careful not to break the yolk. Carefully slide the egg into the well. It will probably overflow a little. Repeat with the second egg and slide it into the second well. Sprinkle herbs, salt and pepper on top of the egg, then sprinkle the cheese over the top. Drizzle 1 tablespoon of heavy cream and Olive Oil over the top. (1/2 to each dish if using 2 dishes.)

Put the dish(es) on a baking pan and slide into the oven. Bake for about 12 to 14 minutes until the egg is set but still slightly runny in the middle, about like a soft boiled egg.

Remove and serve. Beak up the egg and mix it into the sauce and cheese to really mix the flavors. Makes 2 servings.

To make this for more than a couple of people, you can easily double the recipe and use a larger baking dish.

Nutrition Info: 1 egg in half the sauce
Calories: 300 Fat: 23.5 g Net Carbs: 4.6 g Protein: 15.7 g

Mexicali Baked Eggs

This is a variation of the Lasagna Baked Eggs, just with a Mexican flavor. This uses Mexican Chorizo, which is a soft sausage packed with chili sauce in a plastic casing. Don't confuse with Basque Chorizo, which is a harder sausage. (Pictured on page 37.)

1/4 cup Green or Red Enchilada Sauce
1 ounce Mexican Chorizo
1/2 teaspoon crushed Dried Peppers
1/8 teaspoon Cumin
Sprinkle of Mexican Oregano
1/4 teaspoon dried Cilantro
2 tablespoon Queso Fresco, crumbled
2 teaspoons Olive Oil
2 tablespoons Cheddar Jack Cheese
2 Eggs
Salt and Pepper

Preheat oven to 400 degrees F.

In a small oven-proof baking dish or two single-serving casseroles, spray the bottom with cooking spray, then tear the tortilla and layer the pieces on the bottom of the dish, (Split all ingredients if you are making it in two small dishes.) Spoon the enchilada sauce over the tortillas, then sprinkle peppers and cumin on top.

In a small skillet, cook the chorizo until the sauce is melted. Separate into two mounds. Put each mound into the dish to form the base for the eggs. If using a single dish, space these at least three inches apart. Using the back of the spoon, make a well in the middle of the chorizo. Sprinkle a little cheese over the top.

Break an egg in a recipe bowl or small bowl being careful not to break the yolk. Carefully slide the egg into the well. It will probably overflow a little. Repeat with the second egg and slide it into the second well. Sprinkle oregano and cilantro, salt and pepper on top of the egg, then sprinkle the crumbled cheese over the top. Top with shredded cheddar jack cheese. Drizzle 1 tablespoon of heavy cream over the top.

Put the dish(es) on a baking pan and slide into the oven. Bake for about 12 to 14 minutes until the egg is set but still slightly runny in the middle, about like a soft boiled egg. Remove and serve. Beak up the egg and mix it into the sauce and cheese to really mix the flavors.

To make this for more than a couple of people, you can easily double the recipe and use a larger baking dish.

Nutrition Info: 1 egg in half the sauce
  Calories: 300 Fat: 23.5 g Net Carbs: 4.6 g Protein: 15.7 g

Peachy Pecan Pancakes

Although strictly not legal on Atkins phase 2 and phase 3 list, I recently saw a recipe on their site for a dish made with peaches that was fine for phases 2 through 4, so I guess this isn't a hard rule. Use peaches cautiously in your cooking, but a little now and then isn't a bad thing. And this pancake is definitely good! (Pictured on Page 37.)

If you can't get New Hope Mills Sugar Free Pancake Mix, I've put an alternate option below.

2/3 cup New Hope Mills Sugar Free Pancake Mix*
2 tablespoons Vanilla Whey Protein powder (optional)
1/2 teaspoon Baking Powder
1/4 cup diced sugar free canned Peaches, chopped
    or fresh Peach, peeled and chopped
2 tablespoons sugar free Peach Juice
1/4 cup Pecans, chopped
2 tablespoons Coconut Milk unsweetened
1 teaspoon Cinnamon, ground
3 tablespoons Ricotta Cheese, whole milk
1 large Egg
2 tablespoons Butter, melted
2 tablespoons Sugar Substitute

*Or 2/3 cup low carb Baking Mix (or 2 tablespoons Almond Flour and 2 tablespoons Coconut Flour plus 1 egg white) and a pinch of salt

If using fresh peach, cut the peach up and put in a bowl and add 1 tablespoon sugar substitute and mix well. Let it sit, covered in the refrigerator overnight. It should make a juice while it sits.

In a medium bowl, add all the dry ingredients and mix. In another bowl, add egg, butter, coconut milk, peach juice and cinnamon. Stir in ricotta cheese and sugar substitute and stir until blended. Add to the dry ingredients and mix until the batter is combined. If it is too thick, add a little water. It should be easy to spoon and spread on the griddle, but not runny.

Heat a griddle over medium high or an electric griddle to pancake setting. Spray with cooking spray or melt butter on the griddle. Spoon two or three tablespoons onto the griddle and spread to make about a 3" pancake. Repeat with as many cakes as you can fit in and still turn. Let cook about three minutes, then lift the edge to see if the cake is lightly browned. If so, then flip the pancake over and cook another two to three minutes.

Serve with butter and sugar free maple syrup. Makes 5 to 6 pancakes.

Nutrition Info per pancake (assumes 5)
Calories: 103 Fat: 6.5 g Net Carbs: 3.2 g Protein: 7.6 g

Rene Averett

Scottish Eggs

Or possibly Scot's Eggs, but not Scotch Eggs since there isn't a trace of alcohol in them. This is a low carb adaptation of the famous Scottish recipe for these delightfully-tasty sausage and eggs that can be breakfast, lunch or dinner. We used to take them to SCA weekends and they were wonderful when cold or just warmed by the sun as a snack or quick lunch.

To make a meal of them, add a side dish vegetable or a lettuce and tomato salad. Dip them in a little Spicy Mayonnaise sauce or try them with a light curry sauce. They are very versatile. (Pictured on page 37.)

4 medium-sized Eggs, hard boiled	1 large Egg, beaten
1/2 lb ground Sausage	1 teaspoon ground Sage
1/4 teaspoon Salt	1/4 teaspoon Pepper
1 tablespoon chopped Chives	1 teaspoon dried Parsley.
1 tablespoon dried Celeriac (optional)	1 tablespoon Coconut Flour
1/4 cup Almond Flour	

Either boil the eggs and peel them or buy already cooked hard boiled eggs. Preheat oven to 400 degrees. Spray a baking pan with non-stick cooking spray.

Mix the sausage meat and seasonings together. Split meat into four equal balls, then flatten a ball of meat.

On a saucer, spread the coconut flour around. Beat the uncooked egg in a small bowl and use another shallow bowl to put the almond flour. Mix 1/2 teaspoon of dried sage and a pinch or two of salt and pepper into the almond flour.

Take one hardboiled egg, roll it in the coconut flour, then wrap the sausage around it, completely enclosing it. Seal the meat by pressing it with your fingers. Dip the wrapped egg in the beaten egg, then roll in the almond flour. Place on the baking sheet, then repeat this with the other three eggs.

Bake for about 35 minutes. The sausage should be cooked completely through with no pink showing. If there is pink, then cook it a little longer.

Cut the eggs in half, if you wish, and serve with any sauce or dressing you would like or just eat as they are.

Note: You can omit the almond flour and the extra egg if you prefer your eggs without the breading. It will lower the calories and carbs and still be great!

Nutrition Info: per egg (with breading)
Calories: 328 Fat: 25.5 g Net Carbs: 2.5 g Protein: 19.2 g

Nutrition Info: per egg (without breading)
Calories: 270 Fat: 20.8 g Net Carbs: 1.6 g Protein: 16.1 g

Turnip & Sausage Frittata

Usually a frittata is popped into the oven to complete the cooking, but this version is just covered with a lid on the skillet and allowed to finish cooking on the stove for two or three minutes. Turnips, daikon radish or kohlrabi substitute for potatoes or you can use a combination for a bit of variety. Since they take a while to cook, it's best to start with pre-cooked root vegetables rather than try to get them cooked in the pan.

3 Eggs
1 link Italian Sausage, removed from casing
1/4 cup sliced Sweet Peppers
1/2 cup diced Turnips, Daikon Radish or Kohlrabi, pre-cooked
2 tablespoons Pico de Gallo
1 Tablespoon Butter
1Tablespoon Heavy Cream
1/4 cup shredded Parmesan Cheese
1/4 teaspoon Herb Seasoning
Salt and Pepper to taste

In a skillet, cook the sausage until it is browned, separating it into small pieces as you cook. Don't overcook as it will cook more in the frittata.

If the turnips (or other vegetable) aren't already prepared, peel it, dice it and cook in boiling water for about five minutes. The little cubes should be fork tender when you poke them.

Break the eggs into a small bowl, add seasoning, salt, pepper and heavy cream and beat with a fork until well mixed and frothy.

Over medium heat, melt a tablespoon of butter in an omelet skillet, then add the sweet peppers and sauté about five minutes. Add the turnips, Pico de Gallo and sausage and stir to mix into the peppers and butter. Stir the eggs again, then pour into the skillet.

Let cook as for an omelet, allowing the eggs to set, then lift the edges to let the liquid eggs in the middle run underneath to cook. Repeat until most of the liquid egg is set. Turn the heat to low and put a cover over the skillet and let cook about three to five minutes. Check to see if the eggs look set in the middle. If so, then sprinkle the cheese over the top and put the cover back on for two or three minutes. Turn off the heat (if using an electric range, move off the burner) and let sit a couple of minutes.

Cut the frittata in two and serve.

Nutrition Info:
Calories: 388 Fat: 30.5 g Net Carbs: 4.6 g Protein: 21.9 g

Quick Bake French Toast

This is French toast made like a bread pudding. Easy and satisfyingly good. You do need a low carb bread for the base, so refer to the bread section for Irish Soda Bread. Any low carb muffin recipe will also work. Use two regular-sized muffins. (Photo on page 37.)

2 slices (1/12th of loaf each) of New Hope Mills Cranberry
Orange or Blueberry Bread or other low carb bread
    (approx. 2 nc per slice)
2 large Eggs
3 tablespoons Heavy Whipping Cream
2 teaspoons ground Cinnamon
½ teaspoon Vanilla Extract
¼ teaspoon ground Clove

Break bread slices into pieces. In a small bowl, mix eggs, cream, cinnamon, clove and vanilla until well blended. Add bread pieces. Cover with plastic wrap and put in refrigerator for at least one hour (or overnight) to allow bread to soak up the egg mixture.

Preheat oven to 350 degrees (F). Prepare two cassoulet dishes by spraying with cooking spray or butter lightly.

Spoon the French toast mixture evenly into each of the two dishes. Bake for about 25 minutes until the egg bread is firm and lightly browned. Allow to cool for a few minutes, then serve with butter and sugar free pancake syrup.

Makes 2 large servings

Nutrition Info: 1 serving
   Calories: 333.1 Fat: 13.6 g Net Carbs: 3.8 g Protein: 14.8 g

Brunch

Sometimes breakfast turns into lunch, so many of the breakfast choices apply for lunch. But for a true light, but satisfying, lunch, here are several options. They also make a nice, light dinner when you've had a large lunch during the day.

Asian Fusion Dirty Cauli-Rice	46
Asparagus & White Cheese Quiche	47
Bacon, Tomato & Broccoli Pie	48
Chicken à la King	49
Chicken Tacos with Cucumber Salsa	50
Deviled Ham Strata	51
Chicken & Mushroom Crepes	54
Egg Foo Yung	55
Mexican Personal Pizza	56
Sierra Tuna Melt	57
Pollo Pequitos (Little Chickens)	58
Sausage Zucchini Bake	59
Shrimp & Asparagus with Cheese Grits	60
Walnut Chicken Salad	61

Rene Averett

Asian Fusion Dirty Cauli-Rice

One of my favorite meals at the best Asian Bistro in town before it became a sushi place was "Dirty Rice", which is a combination of meat, vegetables and lots of flavor in a fried rice. This version comes close and replaces the rice with cauliflower and daikon riced and cooked to the same texture. Try it before you pooh-pooh it - you'll be surprised at how well the cauliflower substitutes. It is a meal in itself, although you could add a refreshing cucumber, onion, and radish salad with a bit of chilled rice vinegar dressing. For a dinner, add an appetizer. (Photo on page 52.)

1/4 cup finely chopped Onions
1 tablespoons Coconut Oil or Olive Oil
1 Egg, lightly beaten
1 drop Soy Sauce
½ teaspoon Sesame Oil
2 ounces cooked lean boneless Pork, finely chopped
2 ounces Chicken, chopped
1/2 cup small, cooked Shrimp
1/4 cup finely chopped Carrots
1/4 cup Baby Corn, chopped
1/4 cup Chicken Broth
1/4 cup frozen Green Beans, chopped into small pieces
1 1/2 cup frozen or fresh Cauliflower, riced
1/2 cup Daikon, riced
2 Green Onions, chopped
1/2 cup Bean Sprouts
1 tablespoons Soy Sauce

Heat 1 teaspoon oil in wok or rounded side skillet; add chopped onions and stir-fry until onions turn a nice golden color, about 5-7 minutes; remove from wok.

Allow wok to cool for a few minutes. Mix egg with a drop of soy and a drop of oil.

Add 1 teaspoon oil to wok, swirling to coat surfaces; add egg mixture. Immediately swirl egg until egg sets, like an omelet. When egg puffs, flip egg and cook other side briefly; remove from wok, and chop into small pieces.

Heat 1 teaspoon oil in wok; add meats to wok, along with carrots, beans, and cooked onion; stir-fry for 2 minutes.

Add cauliflower, daikon, green onions, bean sprouts and chicken broth. Stir to mix well and continue to stir-fry for 3 minutes, until the liquid is almost gone. Add shrimp and egg and cook another 2 minutes until shrimp are hot. Add soy sauce and stir in. Serve.

Makes 2 servings.

Nutrition Info:
Calories: 233.5 Fat: 9.3 g Net Carbs: 6.8 g Protein: 25.6 g

Asparagus & White Cheese Quiche

Spring is the perfect time to enjoy this crust-less quiche, although you can make it anytime you can get fresh asparagus. Dress it up a little more by adding crumbled bacon to it. It won't add any carbs. (Photo on page 52.)

2 large Egg Yolks
1/4 cup Heavy Cream
1/4 cup Almond Milk
1 teaspoon chopped fresh Tarragon
Dash Nutmeg
Kosher salt and freshly ground Black Pepper
1/4 cup cooked, sliced Asparagus
   (steamed and cut into 1/2 inch slices)
1 cup crumbled fresh Goat Cheese
1 slice thick Bacon, broken into pieces

Position a rack in the center of the oven and preheat oven to 325 degrees (F.)

In a small bowl, add the egg yolks, cream, milk and seasonings and whisk together.

Use 2 one-cup casserole dishes and spray with cooking spray or butter the bottom and sides. Place them on a baking pan. Sprinkle 1/2 the asparagus and goat cheese in each of the dishes, being sure to evenly distribute them.

Whisk the custard again and carefully spoon over the asparagus and cheese. Carefully lift the baking pan and put in the oven. Bake for 25 to 30 minutes. The quiches should be golden brown and slightly puffed. A toothpick inserted in the center should come out clean.

Let cool on a rack for about 10 minutes, then serve warm or at room temperature.

Serves 2.

Nutrition Info for 1 serving
  Calories: 511.7 Fat: 40.9 g Net Carbs: 3.7 g Protein: 31.7 g

Rene Averett

Bacon, Tomato & Broccoli Pie

One of the few recipes in this book that makes more than 2 servings, but I know you will appreciate the leftovers on this one. Use thick sliced bacon, Irish bacon or Montana Red Neck Bacon for best flavor. (Photo on page 52.)

2 slices Montana Cottage Bacon
    Or 4 slices other thick-cut Bacon
1 large Tomato, sliced
1/2 cup Broccoli, chopped
1/2 cup loosely packed Baby Spinach, chopped or torn
1/2 cup Ricotta Cheese, whole milk
2 cups Cheddar Cheese
1 teaspoon Mrs. Dash Tomato, Garlic and Basil Seasoning
3/4 cup Low Carb Flour
1/4 cup Heavy Cream
1/2 cup Water
Dash Salt & Pepper, to taste preference

Heat oven to 425 degrees F. Spray a deep dish pie plate with cooking spray.

Combine the cream and water in a cup and mix. In a small bowl, mix flour, egg, seasonings and 1/2 the cream mixture. Stir well or beat with an egg beater to remove lumps. Add the remaining cream and 1/2 the cheese and mix together. Pour into the pie pan. Bake for 20 minutes.

While crust bakes, put on a pan of water to boil and add the broccoli and let cook for 3 minutes. Drain and run under cool water to stop the cooking. Next, fry the bacon in a skillet until it is crisp. Drain on a paper towel. Crumble or tear bacon into small pieces. In a small bowl, mix together the ricotta cheese, seasonings and chopped spinach.

Remove crust from the oven, spread the ricotta mixture over the top and sprinkle the broccoli and bacon over it. Layer the tomato slices over the bacon and top with the remaining cheese. Put back in the oven for another 15 minutes or until the cheese is lightly browned. Serves 4.

Nutrition Info per slice
Calories: 413.3 Fat 34.8 g: Net Carbs: 4.9 g Protein: 23.5 g

Chicken à la King

What a classic recipe this is! I remember it fondly from my youth and early years after I moved to Los Angeles. It was an inexpensive meal then, but the flavor was fantastic. It's not been around as much in recent years so maybe it's time for a comeback! (Photo on page 52.)

2 tablespoons Butter
1/4 cup small Green Bell Pepper
1 ounce fresh Mushrooms, sliced (about 3 large ones)
2 tablespoons Low Carb Flour
1/8 teaspoon Salt
1/8 teaspoon Pepper
1/4 teaspoon Cayenne Pepper
1/3 cup Heavy Cream
3/4 cup Chicken Broth or Chicken Better than Bullion
3/4 cup cut-up cooked Chicken or Turkey
2 tablespoons dried Tomatoes, cut up & re-hydrated,
    OR 1/4 cup Snow Peas, cut into pieces
1 cup cooked Cauli-rice or 2 slices low carb Bread

Melt 1 tablespoon butter in small sauce pan over medium-high heat. Add bell pepper and mushrooms and sauté until pepper is crisp-tender. Remove from pan and set aside.

Add remaining butter and melt. Stir in flour, salt and pepper. Cook over medium heat, stirring constantly, until flour is bubbly; remove from heat. Stir in milk and broth and cayenne pepper. Heat roux until it bubbles, stirring constantly. Boil and stir 1 minute. Add the bell pepper and mushrooms , then stir in chicken or turkey and tomatoes. Cook until hot. Serve over hot cauli-rice or low carb toast. Serves 2.

For an elegant presentation, use 1/4 sheet of pastry dough and roll out to an 8 x 4 inch rectangle. Cut into two 4x4 inch squares and bake according to the package directions. Move cooked pastry squares to serving plates, cut each diagonally and arrange with long tops to each other to make pasty points. Top with chicken mixture. (Adds 3.75 net carbs to total.)

Nutrition Info per serving without rice or toast (with dried tomatoes)
Calories 491: Fat: 32.7 g Net Carbs 5.3 g: Protein: 42.9 g

Nutrition Info per serving without rice or toast (with snow peas)
Calories 486: Fat: 32.6 g Net Carbs 4.2 g: Protein: 42.7 g

Rene Averett

Chicken Tacos with Cucumber Salsa

Simply wonderful for lunch or for dinner, these tacos and salsa are easy to make. Use precooked chicken and prepare the salsa early. (Photo on page 52.)

Tacos:
1 cup cubed, cooked Chicken breasts
1/4 cup chopped Onions
2 tablespoons chopped Anaheim Green Chile
1 teaspoon Chipotle paste
1/4 teaspoon Cumin
1/4 cup Chicken Bullion
1 teaspoon Olive Oil
1/2 teaspoon minced Garlic
2 low carb Tortillas, 6 inch or Cheese Taco Shells (pg. 142)
1/4 cup shredded Lettuce
1/4 cup shredded Cheddar Cheese
Salt and pepper to taste

Cucumber Salsa:
1 cup chopped Cucumbers
2 tablespoons chopped Chives
2 tablespoons chopped Anaheim chiles
1 tablespoon chopped Cilantro
1 tablespoon Olive Oil
1/2 tablespoon Lemon Juice
1 small clove Garlic, minced
Pinch of Salt

Mix the salsa first: Combine all the salsa ingredients in a small bowl and mix well. Cover with plastic wrap and refrigerate at least one hour.

In a skillet, add 1 teaspoon olive oil and heat to a sizzle. Add minced garlic and onions and stir until onions are just tender. Add the turnips and stir in 1/4 cup chicken bullion

Warm tortillas over an open flame or on a griddle that is on medium high heat. Or wrap in plastic wrap and warm in the microwave for 40 seconds. Or warm in a 400 degree oven for about 10 minutes. If you wish a more traditional taco shell, pour about 1/4 cup oil into a medium sized skillet and heat until it sizzles, then fry each tortilla until lightly browned, then drain on a paper towel. Use immediately before they cool too much and become hard to fold.

Spread 1/2 of the filling down the middle of each tortilla, top with lettuce and cheese. Add a tablespoon of taco sauce. Serve with salsa on the side. Makes 2 servings.

Nutrition Info: Each Serving Taco with toppings
Calories: 275.2 Fat: 11.6 g Net Carbs: 5.6 g Protein: 34.7 g
Salsa- Calories: 33 Fat: 2.4 g Net Carbs: 1.9 g Protein: 0.7 g

Deviled Ham Strata

This is based on a recipe I found in the newspaper many decades ago, but it is still one of the tastiest stratas I've ever had. I have, of course, adapted it to use low carb bread, but it is still wonderfully good. (Photo on page 52.)

4 slices Low Carb Bread
2 oz package Cream Cheese, softened
1 small can of Deviled Ham
1/2 teaspoon Mustard
3 Eggs
1/4 cup Heavy Cream
1/4 cup Water
1/4 teaspoon Salt
1/4 teaspoon Pepper
1/2 cup Cheddar Cheese
1/2 teaspoon Italian Seasoning

Spread 1/2 oz of cream cheese on each slice of the bread. Mix the devil ham with the mustard then spread 1/2 tablespoon of the mixture onto each slice. Spray with baking spray or butter a small baking pan, large enough for a single layer of the bread and 2" to 3" deep. Place the bread slices on the bottom of the pan so they are touching but not overlapping.

In a bowl, mix the eggs, cream, water and seasonings together and stir in the cheese. Pour over the bread in the pan. Cover with plastic wrap and put in the refrigerator to sit for at least one hour. The bread will absorb almost all of the liquid.

Preheat oven to 350 degrees, remove the plastic wrap and bake the strata for about 40 to 50 minutes until it is golden brown and a knife inserted in the middle comes out mostly clean. Let sit about 10 minutes to set, then serve. Makes 4 servings.

Compliment this dish with a fruit salad or a cucumber, tomato and onion salad.

Nutrition Info per serving
Calories: 336.4 Fat: 28.7 g Net Carbs: 3.6 g Protein: 15.2 g

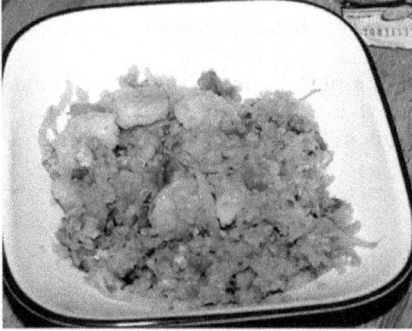

Asian Fusion Dirty Cauli-rice—pg 46

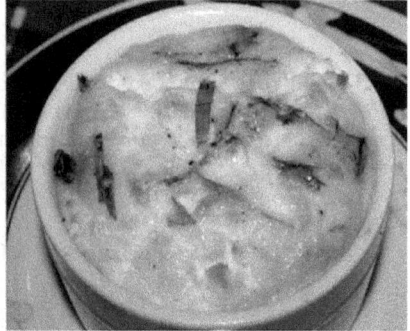

Asparagus & White Cheese Quiche—pg 47

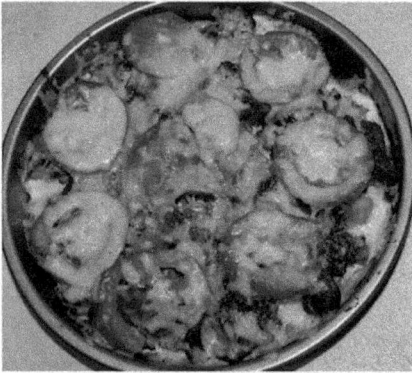

Bacon, Tomato & Broccoli Pie—pg 48

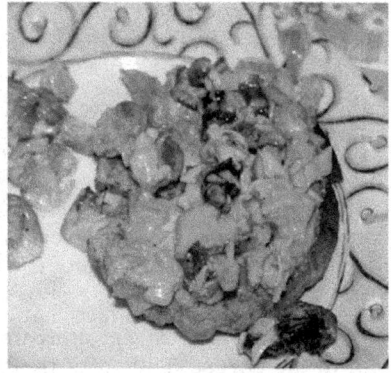

Chicken a la King—pg 49

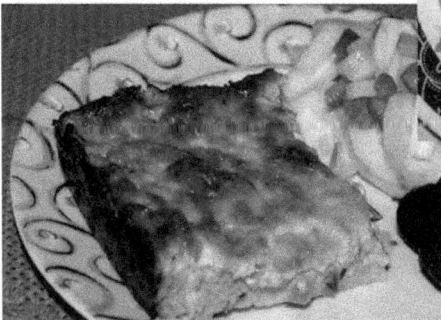

Chicken Tacos with
Cucumber Salsa—pg 50

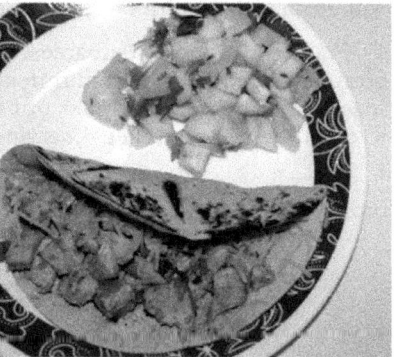

Deviled Ham Strata—pg 51

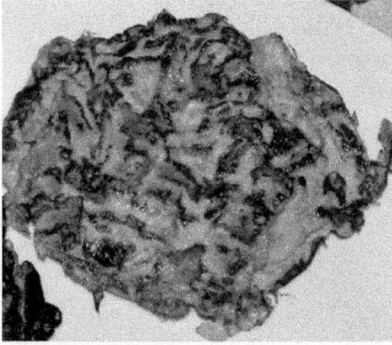

Egg Foo Yung—pg 55

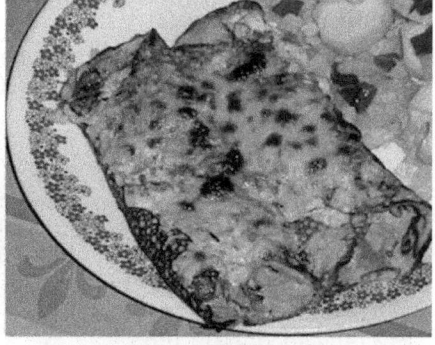

Mushroom & Chicken Crepes—pg 54

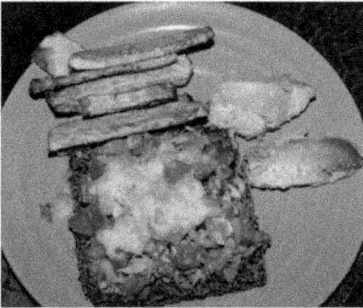

Sierra Tuna Melt—pg 57

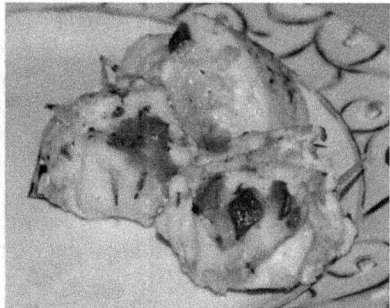

Pollo Pequitos—pg 58

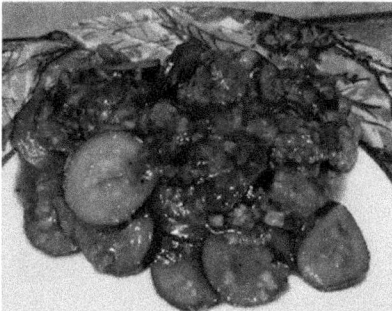

Sausage Zucchini Bake—pg 59

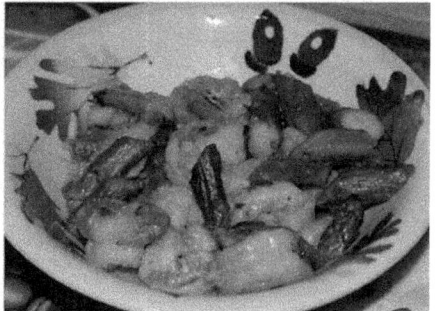

Shrimp & Asparagus Grits—pg 56

Rene Averett

Chicken & Mushroom Crepes

A really tasty crepe filling that goes together easily and looks impressive on the table. Use the basic crepe recipe on page 140 to make your crepes. (Photo on page 53.)

Makes enough filling for 6 crepes. I usually use 2 to 3 per serving.

6 oz. cooked Chicken, cubed or shredded
1 tablespoon Low Carb Flour, such as CarbQuick or Coconut Flour
1/2 cup Heavy Whipping Cream
1/4 cup of Water
2 tablespoons Butter
1 tablespoon Onion, chopped
1/2 teaspoon Italian seasoning
1 cup Mushroom pieces or slices
2 oz. Cream Cheese, cut into cubes
1/3 cup Italian Cheese tri-mix, shredded

In a sauce pan or skillet, melt the butter, add onion and sauté until the onion turns translucent. Add thickener and stir to make a roux. Add the whipping cream and stir well. Remove about 1/2 cup of the sauce. Add the creamed cheese and Italian seasoning and stir until it is mixed well. Then add the chicken and mushrooms and cook until heated thoroughly. Add 1/2 of the Italian cheeses and stir well.

On a plate, place a crepe and put about 2 1/2 tablespoons of filling in the middle. Fold over and secure with a toothpick. Place in a shallow pan or broiler proof dish. Repeat with the remaining crepes. Pour the reserved sauce over the top and sprinkle with the rest of the Italian cheese. Place in the broiler for about 5 minutes. When the top is lightly toasted, remove from the broiler and serve with a salad or fresh vegetables.

Makes 2 to 3 servings

Nutrition Info for 1/6th recipe (filling only)
Calories: 199 Fat: 10.1 g Net Carbs: 2.1 g Protein: 10.4 g

Nutrition Info for 1 crepe (filling and pancake)
Calories: 203 Fat: 11.0 g Net Carbs: 2.9 g Protein: 14.4 g

Egg Foo Yung

This is the Chinese version of an egg fritter and it is great with the brown sauce on it. (Photo on page 53.)

Egg Batter
3 Eggs, lightly beaten
1/3 cup fresh Bean Sprouts
2 tablespoons minced Scallions
2 tablespoons minced Bamboo Shoots
   or Celery or shredded Chinese cabbage
2 Water Chestnuts, minced
1/4 cup slivered, cooked Ham
   or 1/3-1/2 cup Chicken or 1/3-1/2 cup Pork
1/3 teaspoon Soy Sauce
2 tablespoons Coconut Oil (or other cooking oil)

Foo Yung Sauce
1/2 cup Chicken Broth
1 teaspoon Soy Sauce
1/2 teaspoons Sugar Substitute
1/2 teaspoon Vinegar
1 teaspoon Cornstarch
3/4 teaspoons Water

Cut the bean sprouts, celery, water chestnuts and scallions (green onions) into small pieces. Put in a bowl. Add ham, sausage or cooked pork. In a separate bowl, beat eggs and soy sauce together, then mix into the meat and vegetables.

Prepare sauce by mixing chicken broth, soy sauce, and vinegar together. Mix cornstarch and water together. Set aside.

Heat an omelet pan or other small skillet and add a little of the oil to coat the bottom. For small patties, spoon 2 tablespoons of the egg and meat mixture into the skillet. Use a spatula to push any egg that runs out back into the patty, shaping it into a round. Cook over medium high heat for about 1 minute until it is partially set and lightly browned on the bottom. Flip and cook for another minute. Check to see if it is browned, then remove to a warmed plate. Repeat with the remaining egg mixture. To make more at one time, you can use a griddle that will handle about three to four at a time.

For the larger patty, about 4" across, put 1/4 cup of mixture in the middle of the pan and cook the same way, taking about 1 1/2 minutes for each side.

Put the chicken broth mixture into a small pan and bring to a boil, reduce the heat, then add the water and cornstarch mixture and cook until the sauce thickens. Spoon over the egg patties and serve

Makes about six patties

Nutrition Information – 2 small patties or 1 large patty (approx.)
Calories: 136 Fat: 9.4 g Net Carbs: 2.8 g Protein: 9.6 g

Mexican Personal Pizza

Easy to make for 1 or 2 people. This brings Mexican food flavor to a personal "pizza" built on a low carb tortilla. One of my favorite creations. (Photo on page 53.)

Per pizza:

7-inch Low Carb Tortilla
2 tablespoons Black Bean and Corn Salsa or other salsa of choice
2 Sausage Patties, browned and broken into pieces
2 tablespoons Sweet Pepper, diced or sliced thinly
2 tablespoons chopped Onions
1/4 cup Mexican Cheese mix (Cheddar & Jack Cheese)
2 tablespoons Queso Fresco Cheese

Preheat oven to 375 degrees (F) Place a piece of aluminum foil on a baking pan and spray with baking spray.

Put the tortilla on the foil, then top with the salsa. Distribute the sausage and vegetables evenly over the salsa. Sprinkle the cheeses over the top.

Bake for about 15 minutes. Cheeses should be completely melted and possibly light brown.

Cut into wedges and serve. Makes one serving.

Nutrition Info for one:
Calories: 350 Fat 24 g: Net Carbs: 6.9 g Protein: 23.3 g

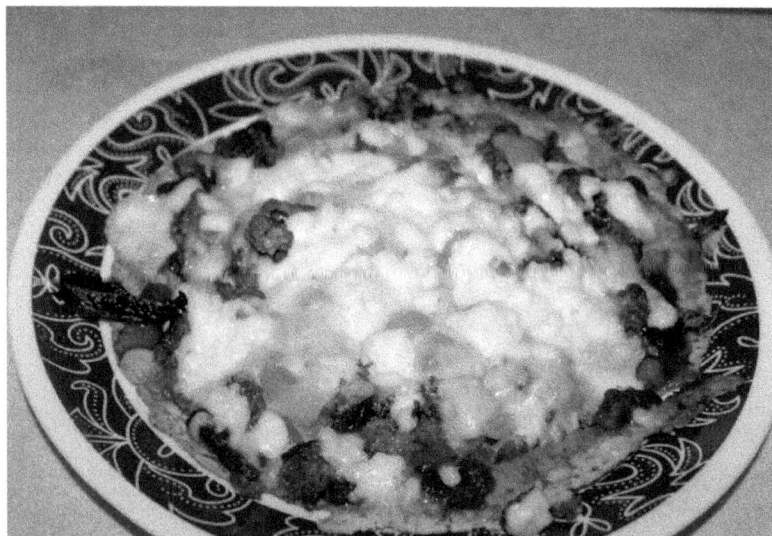

Sierra Tuna Melt

A spiced-up variation on the traditional tuna melt in an open-faced sandwich filled with tuna, tomato, Mexican cheese and spices for a south of the border taste. (Photo on page 53.)

1/4 cup Tuna, drained	1/4 cup small-diced Tomato
2 tablespoons minced Green Onion	Kosher Salt
1 tablespoon chopped Sweet Peppers	1 teaspoon Olive Oil
1/2 teaspoon ground Cumin	1/2 teaspoon dried Oregano
1 tablespoon Mayonnaise	2 tablespoons Queso Fresco
1-1/2 teaspoon White Wine Vinegar	Black Pepper, freshly ground
1/4 cup shredded Cheddar Jack Cheese	

Heat the broiler to high. If you can adjust the rack, position it about 4" from the heat source.

In a medium bowl, combine the tuna, tomato, green onions, peppers, cumin, oregano, mayonnaise, vinegar, olive oil, 1/4 tsp. salt, and a few grinds of pepper.

Cut a square of Focaccia Bread, (page 142) through the middle to make two slices.

Put the bread on a baking sheet or on a sheet of foil on the broiler pan. Broil until lightly toasted, 30 seconds to 1 minute. Watch it closely. Remove the pan from the broiler, flip the bread over, and spread the tuna mixture evenly over each piece.

Crumble the queso Fresco over the tuna, then top with sprinkles of cheddar jack cheese and broil until the cheese is melted and beginning to brown, 2 to 4 minutes, depending on how close your sandwich is to the heat. Serve with sliced avocado and a side salad or vegetable.

Serves 2 lunch sized portions or 1 very hungry person.

Nutrition Info (filling only, see Focaccia Bread for nutrition info) per serving:
Calories:256.3 Fat: 15.8 Net Carbs: 2.2 g Protein: 26.5 g

Note: Net Carbs with bread is 3.3 net carbs. Both sandwiches would be 6.6 net carbs if feeding a larger appetite.

Pollo Pequitos (Little Chickens)

Little rolls of chicken with cream cheese and salsa that make a very nice luncheon for two. (Photo on page 53.)

2 large half Chicken Breasts , no skin
3 oz. Cream Cheese, softened
1/4 cup Green Chile Salsa, Mild or medium
1/4 cup finely chopped Celery (about 2 medium stalks)
1/4 cup Shredded Cheddar & Monterey Jack Cheese
1/4 teaspoon Garlic powder
Dash of Salt and Pepper

You'll need tooth picks to secure the rolls.

If chicken breasts are very thick, cut them in half lengthwise. Pound each potion of chicken with a meat mallet on a cutting board to flatten and shape it into a rectangle as much as possible. Cut the chicken into 1" wide by about half the length of the rectangle strip. (About 1"x3" - if you have a short piece, don't cut it into two pieces.)

Prepare a baking sheet with aluminum foil or a silicone baking mat sprayed with cooking spray. Preheat oven to 350 degrees (F).

Mix the cream cheese with the garlic powder and the shredded cheese. Spread a thin layer of the cream cheese mixture on each strip of chicken, leaving about 1/4 inch on one end free. Brush or use a spoon to spread about 1/2 teaspoon green chili salsa on each strip and sprinkle in the middle with 1/2 teaspoon celery. Roll each chicken strip up toward the ingredient free end to form a roll and secure with a toothpick. Put each on the baking sheet as it is completed.

Brush or spoon any extra salsa over the rolls. Bake for 20 minutes and check for doneness. Continue to cook at 5 minute intervals if they aren't quite done. They won't brown but if you poke the chicken, any juices should run clear. Let cool a few minutes then remove to serving dish. Serve with additional green salsa if you wish.

Makes 2 servings.

Nutrition Info per serving
Calories: 308.5 Fat: 19.2 g Net Carbs: 3.8 g Protein: 30.1 g

Sausage Zucchini Bake

A recipe that was gleaned from the recipe box of a dear friend. She made it for years and I'm not sure where it originated, but it is Italian comfort food and naturally low carb. This makes 4 servings so you have enough for two meals or guests. (Photo on page 53.)

2 cups Zucchini, sliced 1/4 inch
1/2 lb Pork Sausage
1 cup Mozzarella Cheese
1/4 cup Parmesan Reggiano cheese, grated
1 clove Garlic
1/4 cup Onions
1/4 cup chopped Sweet Peppers
1 teaspoon Italian Seasoning
1 cup Pasta Sauce

Wash and slice zucchini into 1/4-inch pieces. Place in pan with enough water to cover. Add chopped garlic and salt. Cook until tender but do not overcook. When done, drain in colander and gently mash to remove as much water as possible. Meanwhile, in a frying pan brown sausage, drain well.

Mix zucchini, sausage and grated mozzarella cheese together, reserving some of the cheese. Put into ovenproof dish leaving room for the juices. Top with spaghetti sauce and remaining mozzarella cheese. Sprinkle Parmesan over top. Bake uncovered at 375 degrees for 25 to 40 minutes or until well browned on top.

Makes 4 servings

Nutrition Info per serving:
Calories: 396 Fat: 31.6 g Net Carbs: 8.3 g Protein: 22.9 g

Shrimp & Asparagus with Cheese Grits

Like many of my recipes, this is adapted from another recipe to make it low carb. The biggest change is to make the grits from cauliflower. Of course, it doesn't taste exactly like southern grits, but it is a good substitute. (Photo on page 53.)

2 tablespoons Butter
1 teaspoon Garlic, minced
3/4 cup Chicken Broth
1 cups riced Cauliflower
1/2 cup riced Daikon
freshly ground Black Pepper
1/2 cup grated Extra-sharp Cheddar
1/4 teaspoon Cayenne Pepper
1/4 teaspoon Hot Sauce (Tabasco or other brand)
1/2 lb. medium Asparagus, sliced diagonally into 1-inch pieces
1/2 lb. large Shrimp, peeled and deveined
1 to 2 Scallions, thinly sliced

Heat 1/2 tablespoon butter in a medium skillet over medium heat. Add the garlic and sliced scallions, then cook about 45 seconds. Add the broth and bring to a boil, then add the riced cauliflower, daikon, and cayenne pepper and stir in. Reduce heat to low, cover, and cook, stirring occasionally, until the mixture thickens and most of the liquid has cooked in, 15 to 20 minutes. Stir in the Cheddar cheese. Season to taste with salt and pepper. Cover and set aside in a warm spot.

Heat 1 tablespoon butter in a 10-inch skillet over medium heat. Stir in asparagus and a little salt. Continue to stir until just tender and slightly browned, 3 to 4 minutes. Add the shrimp and cook until the shrimp is opaque and the asparagus is tender, 2 to 3 more minutes. Reduce the heat to low and add the Worcestershire sauce and hot sauce. Melt the remaining butter into the shrimp and asparagus. Serve the shrimp and asparagus over the grits. Serves 2.

Nutrition Info per serving:
  Calories: 387 Fat: 23.3 g Net Carbs: 6.0 g Protein: 33.5 g

Walnut Chicken Salad

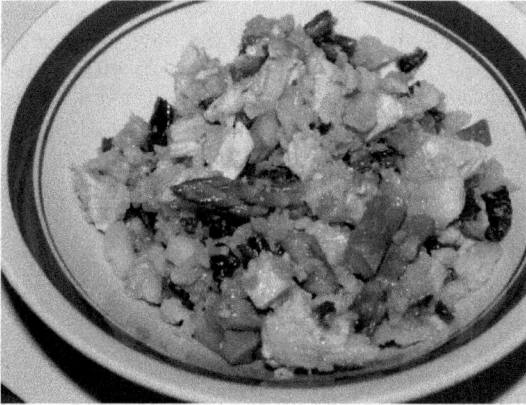

Around my house, all recipes using walnuts get changed to pecans and luckily, the two nuts are pretty much interchangeable. Use whichever one you prefer. You can even use shaved or chopped almonds.

1 cup riced Cauliflower
1/2 cup Chicken Broth
1/4 cup chopped Walnuts
   or Pecans or Almonds
1/4 cup sliced Green Onions

3 stalks Asparagus
1 teaspoon Butter
1 cup diced cooked Chicken
1/4 cup sliced Celery
2 tablespoons diced Red Bell Pepper

Dressing
1 1/2 tablespoons Olive Oil
1/2 tablespoon Soy Sauce
1/2 clove minced Garlic

1 1/2 tablespoons Lemon Juice
1/2 teaspoon Ginger Powder

Make the dressing first: Combine all dressing ingredients into a cruet or dressing bottle, cover and shake well to combine. Refrigerate until ready to use, then shake before serving.

In a large skillet over medium high heat, melt the butter and sauté the nuts until they are browned. Remove to a paper towel on a plate to cool. Add riced cauliflower and daikon to the skillet, then stir in chicken broth. Bring to a boil, then reduce heat to a simmer. Cook for about 30 minutes until most of the liquid is cooked out and the vegetables look fluffy, like rice.

Combine chicken, onions, celery and peppers in a bowl, add nuts and riced mixture and toss together. In a small bowl, combine the dressing ingredients and mix well, then add to the chicken mixture. Refrigerate until ready to serve, allow at least one hour to chill. Makes 2 servings

Nutrition Info per serving:
  Calories: 370.2 Fat 23.3 g: Net Carbs:7.1 g Protein: 30.8 g

Dinners are traditionally the highlight of the day; the time when the family gathers for the evening meal and catching up with each other. A lot of that has drifted away in the past few decades. Even if there are only two people dining, one of these dinner options with a little wine and candlelight can make the evening meal extra special.

Dynamic Dinners

Artichoke & Peppers Chicken Casserole   63
Braised Short Ribs   64
Butternut Squash & Chicken Tostado   65
Chicken Cordon Bleu   66
Chicken Provolone Blanca   69
Rene's Coconut Shrimp   70
Cranberry Mustard Baked Salmon   71
Italian Meatloaf for Two   72
Lasagna Carbonara   73
Rene's Pasta Sauce From Scratch   74
Orange Chicken with Bean Sprouts   75
Parmesan Crusted Chicken   76
Chicken Angelica   77
Peanut Curried White Fish   78
Pecan Crusted Chicken   79
Pork, Butternut & Apple Sauté'   80
Pumpkin Shrimp Curry   81
Salmon Cakes With Dill Sauce   82
Creamy Dill Sauce   83
Feline Version   83
Irish Style Salmon With Bacon and Cabbage   86
Salsa Chicken   87
Crab Stuffed Cod   88
Quick Poached White Fish   89
Scalloped Chicken & Turnips   90
Simple Salisbury Steak   91
Pork Chile Verde   92
Tempura Cod and Vegetables   93
Tempura Batter   94

Artichoke & Peppers Chicken Casserole

Another adapted recipe with my own spin on it. I find the cauliflower and daikon radish combination to be really tasty. You can use all cauliflower if you prefer. The taste on this is unusual and very good. If you can prepare this the day before and let it sit in the 'fridge overnight, the flavors blend better. Add the Parmesan just before putting it under the broiler. (Photo on page 67.)

1 cup Cauliflower, riced
1/4 cup Daikon Radish, riced
3/4 cup Chicken Broth
3/4 cup diced, cooked Chicken
1/2 Red Bell Pepper, roasted or 2 Mini Peppers
2 tablespoons chopped Olives
1/4 cup Low Carb Italian Salad Dressing
1/4 cup shredded fresh Parmesan Cheese
1/4 cup Artichoke Hearts, sliced or chopped
1 tablespoons chopped fresh Parsley
1 teaspoon Garlic Powder or fresh Garlic
Salt and Pepper to taste

Use your food processor to chop the cauliflower and daikon. Pulse a few times until it the size of rice.

Cook cauliflower and daikon in a large deep-sided skillet, preferably one that go into the oven safely, with the chicken broth and seasonings. Cook until tender, about 20 minutes.

Meanwhile roast the peppers under the broiler until just lightly browned and tender. Check frequently so they don't burn. Chop peppers into small pieces.

Add chicken, roasted peppers, olives and salad dressing to the pan and mix well. Cover and continue to cook over low heat for 5 to 10 minutes or until it is thoroughly heated, stirring occasionally. If your skillet isn't oven-safe, pour the mixture into an ungreased 1-quart casserole. Sprinkle with Parmesan cheese.

Broil 4 to 6 inches from heat for 1 to 2 minutes or until cheese is melted. Sprinkle with parsley.

Makes two servings.

Nutrition Info per serving:
  Calories: 308 Fat 9.1 g: Net Carbs:5.4 g Protein: 45.1 g

Braised Short Ribs

Easy to make and melt-in-your-mouth tender, these short ribs have all the flavor and not as many carbs. The vegetables in this are golden beets, which have a less earthy flavor than the red beet, red onions and celery. (Photo on page 67.)

4 Beef Short Ribs (with bones) - about 1 1/2 lbs
1 Golden Beet, medium
1 Red Onion, medium
2 stalks Celery, cut into 1" pieces
1 Turnip, medium
1/2 cup Beef Bullion
1/2 cup Red Wine (Merlot or Cabernet Sauvignon)
1/2 cup Low Carb Flour or Coconut Flour
2 tablespoons Olive Oil
1 teaspoon Seasoning Salt
1/2 teaspoon Garlic Powder
1/2 teaspoon Black Pepper, ground

Preheat oven to 325 degrees (F)

Peel the beet and turnip and cut into cubes. Peel the onion and slice it.

In a pie pan, mix the flour with the seasoning salt and garlic powder. Dredge the short ribs in the flour.

In a Dutch oven or heavy oven-ready pan, heat 1 tablespoon olive oil until hot. Add the onions and vegetables and cook until just browned. Remove to a plate. Add the remaining oil, then add the short ribs and brown on all sides, about three minutes a side. When browned, add the beef bouillon and wine and stir. Then add the vegetables back in.

Cover the pot with an oven-proof lid or heavy foil and put in the preheated oven. Cook for 2 hours. Short ribs will be tender and delicious.

Serves 2.

Nutrition Info:
Calories: 448 Fat: 24.4 g Net Carbs: 8.6 g Protein: 35.7 g

Butternut Squash & Chicken Tostado

Butternut is a great vegetable for many dishes. It is lower in carbs than a sweet potato and stands in nicely in many dishes. This one really features it in a flavorful medley. (Photo on page 67.)

1/4 cup Onions, chopped
1/4 cup Butternut Squash, cut into 1/4 -inch cubes
1/4 cup diced Bell Pepper
1/2 cup Cooked Chicken, shredded or diced
1/2 tablespoon Olive Oil
2 tablespoons Taco Sauce
2 low carb Flour Tortillas
1/2 cup shredded Monterey Jack Cheese
Fresh Cilantro leaves, torn
2 cups shredded Lettuce
1/2 Hass Avocado, cut into slices
2 tablespoons Pico de Gallo or Salsa

Preheat oven to 375 degrees (F.)

Use a tostada mold to make the tortilla shells or turn a muffin pan upside down and arrange the tortillas over the cup and press down to make a well in the tortilla. If the tortilla doesn't bend easily, heat it over a burner for about 30 seconds until it softens or warm in the microwave for about 20 seconds. Bake the shell for 8- 10 minutes until it is lightly browned. Let cool.

In a large skillet, heat the oil, then add the onions and bell pepper and sauté for about 1 minute over medium high heat. Add the squash cubes and the chicken and continue to cook for about 5 minutes. Add the taco sauce, cover the pan, reduce the heat to medium and cook for another 5 minutes. (If the vegetables are getting dry, add a little water to the pan.)

Put lettuce in the bottom of the tortilla shell, then spoon 1/4 of the filling into the shell, making sure to distribute it into the points. Top with shredded cheese and put a slice of avocado on top of each point of the tostada. Spoon the Pico de Gallo or salsa into the middle. Serve with a low carb chipotle ranch dressing if you like.

Makes 2 servings

Nutrition Info per serving:
Calories: 191.2 Fat: 19.9 g Net Carbs: 10.2 g Protein: 25.5 g

TIP: Want to reduce your carbs a little? Omit the tortillas and just eat as a salad. This reduces the meal by 3 net carbs and 60 calories. To make this vegetarian, omit the chicken.

Chicken Cordon Bleu

No doubt about it, this is a classic recipe and a wonderful way to prepare chicken. Being fond of cranberries, I used cranberry mustard in it, which brings a little tanginess to the dish. But you can use Dijon mustard if you prefer. (Photo on page 67.)

2 half Chicken Breasts , no skin
4 Deli-Ham slices
2 oz. Gruyere cheese or Swiss cheese, sliced thinly
1/8 teaspoon Garlic powder
1/8 teaspoon Paprika
Dash of Salt and Pepper
2 tablespoons Butter
2 tablespoons Cranberry Mustard
2 tablespoons Almond Flour

Preheat oven to 350 degrees (F.)

Using a meat mallet, pound chicken breasts until they are flattened into a rectangle. Place 2 pieces of ham on each chicken breast, then top with Swiss cheese and spread cranberry mustard over the cheese. Roll the chicken up and secure with toothpicks. Mix garlic powder, salt and pepper with almond flour. Melt butter in a bowl wide enough to accommodate the chicken rolls. Dip the chicken rolls into the butter, then roll in the almond flour to lightly coat.

Spray a small pan with baking spray and place the chicken rolls in the pan. Drizzle any extra butter over the top.

Bake for 20 to 30 minutes until any juices from the chicken are clear. Let rest about five minutes, then serve.

Makes 2 servings.

Nutrition Info per serving made with almond flour
    Calories:434.8 Fat: 16.3 g   Net Carbs: 2.5 g   Protein: 40.1 g

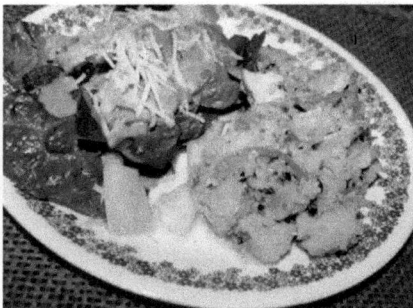

Artichoke & Pepper Chicken Casserole—pg 63

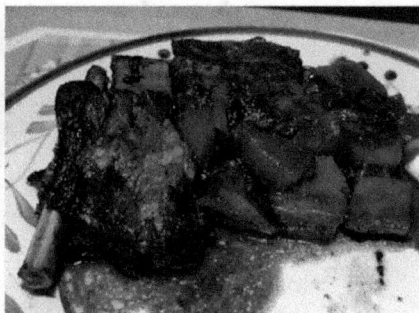

Braised Short Ribs—pg 64

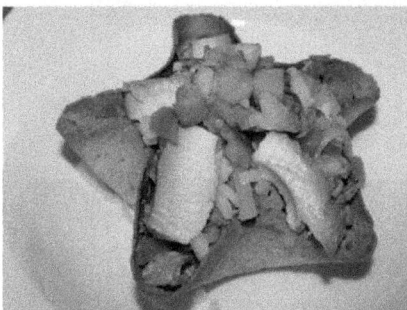

Butternut Squash & Chicken Tostado—pg 65

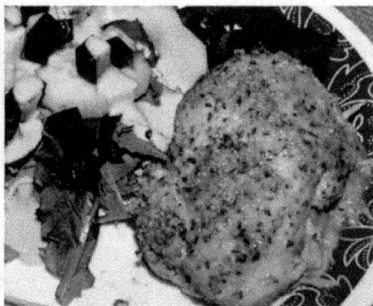

Parmesan Crusted Chicken—pg 76

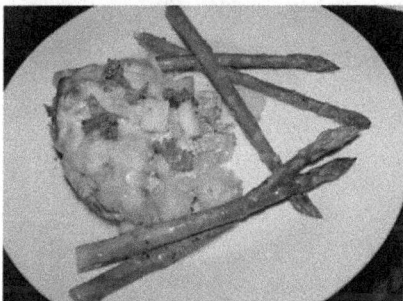

Chicken Provolone Blanca—pg 69

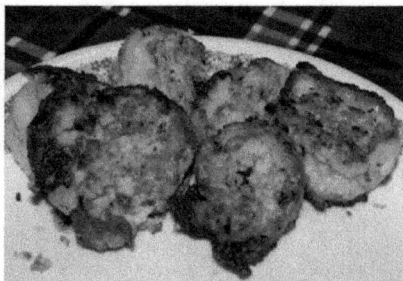

Rene's Coconut Shrimp—pg 70

Cranberry Mustard Baked Salmon—pg 71

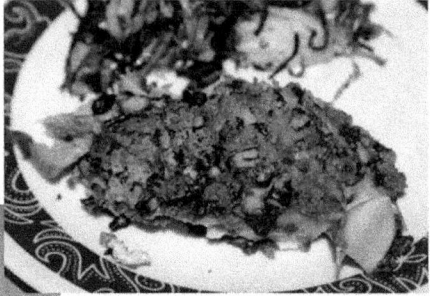

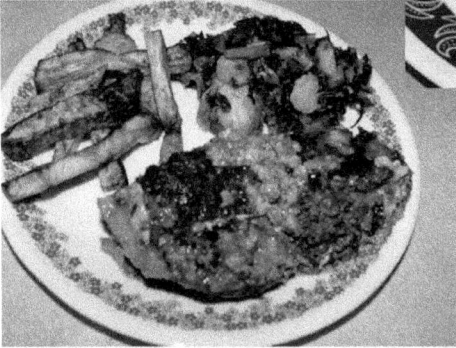

Italian Meatloaf —pg 72

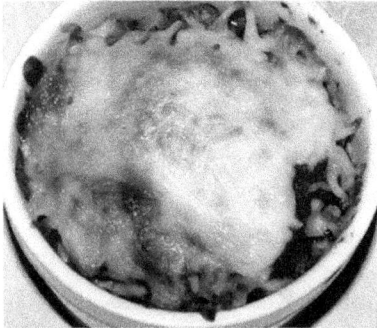

Lasagna Carbonara—pg 73

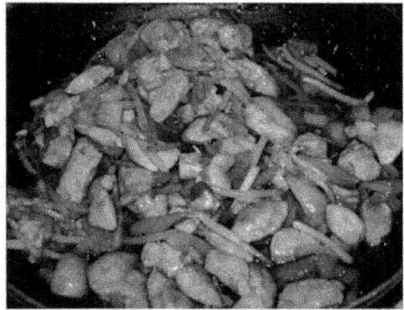

Orange Chicken —pg 75

Parmesan Crusted Chicken—pg 76

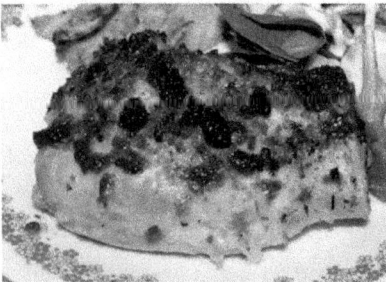

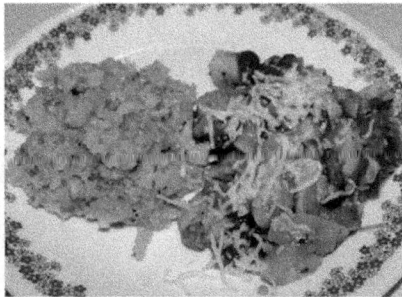

Chicken Angelica—pg 77

Chicken Provolone Blanca

Simple to prepare, yet elegant, dish with a light flavor. I designed this to feature kohlrabi, an infrequently used vegetable that is delicious. If you like the taste of broccoli stems, then you will likely enjoy the slightly milder flavor of kohlrabi. (Photo on page 67.)

2 skinless boneless Chicken Half Breasts
Pepper & Seasoning Salt
1 teaspoon Garlic, minced
1 tablespoon Olive oil
1 tablespoons Butter
1 cup Kohlrabi or Broccoli
   Stems, 1/2" diced
1 tablespoons chopped Parsley

2 tablespoons Almond Flour
1 Egg, separated
1 tablespoon Sherry Wine
1/3 cup sliced fresh Leek
2 slices Provolone Cheese

White sauce
1 tablespoon Butter
1/4 cup Water
1/2 teaspoon Chicken Bullion

3 tablespoons Heavy Cream
Salt & Pepper to taste

Make the white sauce by melting the butter in a small pan over medium heat. Stir in the cream and water and bullion and stir until blended. Cook over medium heat until the sauce comes to a slow boil. In a small bowl, beat the egg yolk, then add a tablespoon of the sauce and stir until it is blended. Add another tablespoon of cream sauce and stir it in. Add the egg yolk blend to the sauce gradually and stir it in as you do. Reduce heat to a simmer. Add a bit of pepper. When the consistency is a thick sauce, remove from heat and set aside

Preheat oven to 350 degrees (F.)

Put the almond flour, seasoning salt and pepper in a shallow pan or bowl. Beat the egg white with a fork in a shallow bowl. Coat the chicken with egg white, then roll in the almond flour, shaking off any excess. This should be a light coating rather than breading.

In a medium skillet, add oil and heat. Brown the chicken pieces on both sides until lightly browned. Transfer to a small baking dish. Add butter to the skillet and melt over medium heat. Sauté the leeks until just lightly browned and limp, then add the kohlrabi, a tablespoon or two of water and cook until the kohlrabi is fork tender. Stir in the sherry and cook another 2 minutes. Add the cream sauce and mix well.

Top each chicken piece with a slice of Provolone cheese. Bake for 30 minutes. Arrange the chicken and vegetables on the plate and add a bit of parsley for color. Serves two.

Nutrition Info per serving
Calories: 524 Fat: 38 g Net Carbs: 6.7 g Protein: 33.4 g

Rene's Coconut Shrimp

One of the wonderful shrimp dishes that are on many restaurant menus and just needed to be adapted to low carb. I use unsweetened dried coconut flakes from Bob's Red Mill, but you need to soak them in warm water or coconut milk to reconstitute a little and revitalize the flavor. If you buy unsweetened peaches in sugar free syrup, you can use that for the peach syrup. (Photo on page 67.)

1/2 pound large Shrimp, peeled and deveined
1/4 cup Coconut Flour
1/2 teaspoon Salt
1/4 teaspoon Cayenne Pepper
1/2 cup flaked Unsweetened Coconut
1/4 cup Warm Water or Coconut Milk
1 tablespoon Sugar Substitute
2 Egg Whites, beaten

Rene's Dipping Sauce
1/4 cup Sugar Free Peach Syrup
2 tablespoons Water
1 tablespoons Vinegar
1 teaspoon Soy Sauce
2 tablespoons Brown Sugar Substitute or Sugar Free Maple Syrup
1 teaspoon Cornstarch

Preheat oven to 350 degrees (F.) Spray a baking pan or cookie sheet with baking spray.

Clean and devein shrimp and dry on a paper towel. In a small bowl, put the flaked coconut, warm water and sugar substitute to soak for at least 5 minutes. This will sweeten the coconut and soften it a bit.

Prepare the dipping sauce while oven heats. In a sauce pan, add all the ingredients and stir until mixed, then heat over medium heat until the sauce thickens. Turn off heat.

Beat egg whites until foamy, but not stiff. Mix coconut flour, salt and Cayenne pepper together in a small bowl or tin. Drain coconut and put in a separate pan. Roll a shrimp in the flour mixture, then dip in the egg white and roll in the coconut to coat it. Put on prepared baking tin. Repeat with the remaining shrimp until all are coated.

Bake about 10 minutes, then turn the shrimp over and bake another 8 to 10 minutes until shrimp are cooked through. Be careful to not overcook the shrimp.

Serve with the dipping sauce. Serves two.

Nutrition Info per serving:
  Calories: 388 Fat: 55 g Net Carbs: 10.7 g Protein: 27.8 g

Cranberry Mustard Baked Salmon

I fell in love with this the first time I tried it. It's an absolutely delicious way to prepare salmon. I used low carb Irish soda bread crumbs and Beaver's Cranberry mustard. You could also use 2 tablespoons of almond flour to substitute for the bread crumbs. (Photo on page 68.)

2 tablespoons Butter, salted
1 1/2 tablespoons Cranberry Mustard
2 tablespoons low carb Bread Crumbs
2 tablespoons Pecans, chopped
2 filets Salmon - 4oz each

Preheat oven to 400 degrees (F).

Rinse salmon off and pat dry with a paper towel. Melt butter, add cranberry mustard and stir. In a recipe bowl, mix low carb bread crumbs and pecans.

Spread butter mixture over the top of the salmon using a spoon to evenly coat it. Sprinkle the pecan and crumbs topping over the filets and press it gently into the coating.

Bake for 12 to 15 minutes until the salmon flakes easily with a fork.

Serves 2.

Nutrition Info: (estimated - will vary with bread crumbs)
  Calories: 348 Fat: 21.5 g Net Carbs: 5.6 g Protein: 23 g

Rene Averett

Italian Meatloaf for Two

We often overlook meatloaf when planning menus, but it is a great way to use ground beef and add a bit of sausage if you like, in a wonderfully satisfying meal. Add the Italian seasonings and it's a bit like eating an Italian meatball. (Photo on page 68.)

8 oz. Ground Beef
1 tablespoon Dried Onion Flake or 2 tablespoons chopped onion
1 cup Mozzarella cheese
2 tablespoons grated Parmesan Cheese
1 teaspoon Seasoning Salt
1/4 teaspoon Ground Thyme
1/4 teaspoon Pepper
1 Egg
1 slice low carb Bread Roll, crumbled or processed to crumbs*
1 cup fresh Spinach, sliced or torn into small pieces
1/2 cup Pasta Sauce, (look for 3 to 5 carbs per serving)
2 tablespoons Cream Cheese, softened (optional)

* I used 1/2 of a low carb sandwich roll

Lightly spray a small loaf pan or casserole dish with cooking spray. Preheat oven to 365 degrees F.

In a small bowl, combine all the ingredients and mix well. Put into baking pan and shape into a loaf.

Bake for 30 to 35 minutes until the meat is completely cooked and the top is browned. Let cool and set for about 5 minutes before serving.

Nutrition Info per serving
 Calories: 407 Fat: 11.3 g Net Carbs: 5.6 g Protein: 42.4 g

Lasagna Carbonara

I used Classico Vodka pasta sauce for this recipe. You can also use Mario Battali's Vodka pasta sauce. They are the lowest I've found in carbohydrates. I've tried pizza sauce, which is about the same in carbs, but not as flavorful or as thick. Or you can make your own sauce from scratch, if you prefer. (Photo on page 68.)

4 tablespoons Low Carb Pasta Sauce
2 tablespoons Ricotta Cheese, whole milk
1/4 cup shredded Mozzarella Cheese
1/4 lb Ground Beef, cooked
4 tablespoons Bacon Pieces
1 tablespoons sliced Olives
1 tsp Italian Seasoning
1/2 tsp Garlic
1/2 tablespoon dried Chives
1 medium Zucchini, cut into long flat strips*
1/4 teaspoon Dried Chile flakes

* To cut the zucchini, trim the ends, then lay zucchini on its side and slice lengthwise into ¼ inch by length. Heat a sauce pan of water to boiling. Cook zucchini noodles in the hot water about 3 minutes. Drain. Can be cooked ahead of time.

Cook the ground beef in a skillet or use leftover ground beef or a pre-cooked patty broken into pieces. I used a pre-made grilled hamburger patty for this.

Add the Italian seasoning, dried chives and garlic to the ricotta cheese.

Preheat oven or toaster oven to 365 degrees F.

Spray a two cup casserole dish or 2 one cup ramekins with cooking spray. Layer the ingredients similar to this -- split the amounts in half for the ramekins - amount noted in (parentheses):
Pasta sauce - 1 (1/2) tablespoon spread on the bottom
Zucchini slices – 1/2 (1/4) slices - cut and arranged to fit
Ricotta cheese - 2 (1) tablespoons, spread over the zucchini
Sliced olives - 1 (1/2) tablespoon arranged evenly
Dried Chile flakes - 1/4 (1/8) sprinkled over it
Hamburger pieces - 1/2 (1/4) spread over the top
Bacon pieces - 4 (2) tablespoons, sprinkled over the hamburger
Mozzarella cheese - 2 (1) tablespoons sprinkled
Zucchini slices - 1/2 (1/4) arranged over the cheese
Pasta sauce - 1 (1/2) tablespoon spread over the zucchini
Hamburger pieces - Remaining 1/2 (1/4) spread over the top
Zucchini slices - Remaining 2 (1) pieces

Mozzarella cheese - 2 (1) tablespoons

Bake this in an oven or toaster oven preheated to 365 degrees F. for 18 to 20 minutes.

You can also cook this in the microwave. Allow 1 to 1 1/2 minutes in a high powered oven to get completely hot.

Tip: The dish can be prepared ahead of time, covered with plastic wrap, and put in the 'fridge until ready to cook.

Nutrition Info per serving
  Calories: 232.5 Fat:11.6 g Net Carbs: 4.3 g Protein: 22.5 g

Rene's Pasta Sauce From Scratch

1/2 cup canned Tomatoes, with juice
2 tablespoons Onion, chopped
1 teaspoon Garlic, minced
1/2 teaspoon Garlic Powder
1 teaspoon Oregano
1 teaspoon Basil
1 teaspoon Italian seasoning
1 teaspoon Butter
1/4 cup Water
1 teaspoon Sugar Substitute
2 tablespoons dry Red Wine

Mix all ingredients in a sauce pan and cook over medium heat until the sauce reduces to the desired thickness. It will make about one cup of sauce. Try to make the sauce at least one day prior to when you want to use it to allow the flavors to intensify.

Nutrition Info per recipe:
  Calories: 100 Fat: 4.2 g Net Carbs: 7.8 g Protein: 1.8 g

Orange Chicken with Bean Sprouts

Orange isn't high on the list of okay foods if you're trying to stay really low carb. By using the combination of a little orange juice and orange extract, it brings the orange flavor to the dish without adding too many carbohydrates. If you can't find sugar free honey, then omit it and add one tablespoon of sugar substitute. (Photo on page 68.)

1/2 pound boneless, skinless Chicken Breasts
1 tablespoons Butter or Coconut Oil
2 tablespoons Orange Juice* (See note)
1/2 teaspoon Orange Extract
1 tablespoons Water
1/2 tablespoon Orange Zest
1 1/2 tablespoons Oyster Sauce
1 tablespoons Sugar Free Honey
1/2 teaspoon Brown Sugar Substitute
1/2 teaspoon Cornstarch
1 teaspoons minced Ginger
1/4 Onion, sliced
1/8 teaspoon Red Pepper Flakes (optional)
1/2 cup Bean Sprouts (optional)
1 tablespoons chopped Green Onions, including the green tops

Partially freeze the chicken to make it easier to cut, then cut it into bite-sized pieces. Dry chicken with paper towels

Prepare the sauce ingredients by mixing the orange juice and zest, the orange extract, brown sugar substitute, ginger and pepper flakes, then set aside. In a small bowl, add the water and cornstarch and mix well. Set aside.

Heat the butter or oil in a large skillet or wok until hot. Add half of the chicken and cook until brown. Remove to a paper towel covered plate, then cook the rest of the chicken and drain on paper towel. Small batches help control the temperature of the pan so the chicken will cook more evenly.

In the same skillet or wok with the pan drippings from the chicken, add the onions and a little more oil, if needed, and stir fry until tender, then spoon the onions out to the paper towel. Add the sauce mix to the wok, then the honey and stir together. Add the cornstarch and water to thicken. Use a wooden spoon to stir well and scrape the bits of meat that have stuck to the pan.

Toss in your chicken and onions and heat it through. Add bean sprouts and green onions and cook one more minute. Serves 4.

Nutrition Info per serving
Calories: 192.5 Fat: 5.6g Net Carbs: 6.3 g Protein: 6.4 g

Parmesan Crusted Chicken

My adaptation of a popular recipe for mayonnaise and parmesan encrusted chicken. This is so easy to make and tastes so good. It's a quick go-to meal anytime. Almond flour or ground almonds make a great substitute for bread crumbs in this and many other recipes. (Photo on page 68.)

1/4 cup Mayonnaise
2 tablespoons grated Parmesan cheese
2 Chicken Breasts, about 4 oz. each
2 teaspoons Italian Seasoning
2 teaspoons low carb Bread Crumbs or Ground Almonds

Preheat oven to 425 degrees (F.). Spray a small tin or baking sheet with cooking spray.

In a small bowl, mix the mayonnaise with Italian seasonings and grated cheese. Arrange chicken on baking sheet. Spread the mayonnaise mixture over the chicken, then sprinkle with bread crumbs or ground almonds.

Bake until chicken is thoroughly cooked and juices run clear, about 25 minutes. Serve with a sprig of fresh parsley for color.

Nutrition Info per serving
  Calories: 350 Fat: 25.4 g Net Carbs: 0.4 g Protein: 28.4 g

Chicken Angelica

An easy, elegant chicken dish that was originally made with angel hair pasta, but for low carb, we're substituting yellow squash. You could also use zucchini cut into thin strips or spaghetti squash. Using pre-cooked chicken speeds this dish along. (Photo on page 68.)

1 large Chicken Breast, cooked and cut into pieces
1 cup Yellow Crookneck Squash, diced
1 cup canned Tomatoes
2 teaspoons Italian Seasonings
1 teaspoon Oregano
1/4 teaspoon ground Pepper
1/4 cup Bell Peppers chopped
1 cup shredded Mozzarella Cheese
2 tablespoons Parmesan Cheese, grated
1 tablespoon Olive Oil
1/4 cup Mushrooms, fresh, sliced or chopped

In a skillet, add the olive oil and stir fry the mushrooms and bell peppers. Add the tomatoes and seasonings, then add 1/4 cup of water and the diced squash. Bring to a boil, then reduce to a simmer and cook until the squash is just fork tender. If it gets too dry add a little water. When the squash is done, add the chicken and half the mozzarella, stir it well and cook for another 5 minutes.

Serve on the plates and top with the remaining mozzarella.

Makes 2 servings.

Nutrition info per serving:
Calories: 387 Fat: 17.3 g Net Carbs: 8.8 g Protein: 45.1 g

Peanut Curried White Fish

With curries, you're either a fan or you aren't. So for the fans, this is a great fish dish that combines the curry flavors with butternut squash. I like to use the paste cubes to make the curry since it gives a stronger flavor than the dry spices seem to do. But use whatever method you prefer. (Photo on page 84.)

2 Fish Filets (cod or other white fish,) about 1 inch thick
1 square S&B Golden Curry Sauce Mix (1/5 pkg)
1/4 teaspoon Dried Red Chili Pepper
1/2 cup Butternut or Acorn Squash
1 teaspoon Peanut Butter
1/3 cup Coconut Milk
Salt and Pepper

Preheat oven to 350 degrees F. (180 degrees C.)

Cut squash into small cubes, place into a small microwavable bowl and microwave for 2 minutes, stir and microwave another 2 minutes. Check to see if they are fork-tender, easily pierced with a fork. You want them firm, but not hard.

In a pan, put 1 square of the Golden Curry paste and turn on low heat to melt it. Add peanut butter and coconut milk. Stir and cook until blended. It will be thick. Add a little water to make it an easily spreadable consistency.

Oil or spray a baking pan and put about a tablespoon of the curry in it. Place the fish filets on top, add salt and pepper. Reserve another tablespoon of the curry, then spread the rest of the curry over the top of the fish, then pile the squash on top of that and spread the rest of the curry over the squash.

Cover with foil and bake for 15 minutes. Remove the foil and bake another 5 minutes. Remove to serving plates and use the spatula or a spoon to scoop up the curry sauce and drizzle over the fish on the plate.

Makes 2 servings

Nutrition Info per serving:
Calories: 218.4 Fat: 6.4 g Net carbs: 8.5 g Protein: 27 g

Pecan Crusted Chicken

Easy to prepare, the chicken is moist and tender inside the pecan crust. This is a quick to make favorite. (Photo on page 84.)

2 skinless, boneless 1/2 Chicken Breasts
1 tablespoons Sugar Free Maple Syrup
1/2 cup chopped Pecans or Walnuts
1 1/2 tablespoons Almond Flour
1/2 teaspoon Salt
1 tablespoons Butter
1 tablespoon Coconut Oil

Preheat oven to 350 degrees F.

On parchment paper or in a tin pan, combine pecans, flour, and salt.
Brush chicken breasts all over with syrup. Roll chicken breasts in nut mixture to completely coat.

In a cast iron or other oven proof skillet, cooking over medium heat, melt butter and stir in the vegetable oil. Add chicken, and cook for 10 minutes until chicken is lightly browned on both sides.

Put in the oven and cook an additional 10 minutes until the chicken is cooked completely and is fork tender.

Nutrition Info per serving
Calories: 419.5 Fat: 6.6 g Net Carbs: 2.0 g Protein: 23.6 g

Pork, Butternut & Apple Sauté'

A beautiful, elegant dish, this recipe is a little high on both carbs and calories, but it is well worth the small bit of indulgence to enjoy it now and then. (Photo on page 84.)

3 tablespoon Butter	1 teaspoon Olive Oil
1 tablespoon fresh Parsley	1/4 medium Onion
2 Boneless Pork Ribs	2 tablespoons Cider Vinegar
or an 8 oz. Pork Tenderloin	2 tablespoons Water
1/4 Apple, cubed	1 1/2 teaspoon Ginger, grated
1/2 cup Butternut Squash	Salt & Pepper

Cut the butternut squash into 1" cubes. Cut an apple into quarters, then cut one quarter into 1" cubes. Put the rest in a plastic bag to use for another meal. Peel and cut an onion into quarters and cut one quarter into pieces. Put the rest away.

Slice the pork into four or five pieces and season with salt and pepper. Set aside for the moment.

Over medium heat, melt 1 tablespoon of butter and a teaspoon of oil in a skillet. Add the butternut squash and season with a little salt and pepper. Sauté until they're browned and all sides, as much as possible. This should take about 10 to 12 minutes. Remove to a bowl.

Add another tablespoon of butter to the pan, then add the onions and apples. Season with a bit of salt. Cook, stirring frequently, until both the onions and the apples are browned. Stir in ginger, 1 tablespoon cider vinegar and 1 tablespoon water. Remove the pan from the heat and use a wooden spoon or spatula to scrape the browned bits on the bottom of the pan. Remove to the same bowl as the squash.

Turn the heat up to medium high, add the last of the butter and 1 teaspoon of oil to the pan and heat to sizzling. Add the pork in a single layer and cook until browned on all sides, turning a couple of times. This will take about five minutes. Remove the pork to a plate. To the pan, add the remaining cider vinegar and water and stir well, loosening the bits stuck to the pan. Add the squash, onions and apples back to the pan and stir, cooking for about three to five minutes to reheat.

Arrange the pork on the plate and top with the squash mixture. Add a bit of fresh parsley for color, if you like. Serves two.

Nutrition Info per serving:
Calories; 595.2 Fat: 21 g Net Carbs: 9.5 g Protein: 28.1 g

Pumpkin Shrimp Curry

Anytime you cook with curry and butternut squash, you're going to have a taste-buds-tingling, but slightly higher carb'd, dish so be sure to plan for it in your meal plan. It's worth it for a special treat. (Photo on page 84.)

1 tablespoons Olive Oil	1/4 medium Onion, chopped
1/4 cup Pumpkin Puree	1 tablespoons Garlic Ginger Paste
1/3 cup Chicken Broth	1/4 cup Unsweetened Coconut Milk
1 square Golden Curry	2 drops Lime Juice
1/2 cup Butternut Squash	2/3 cup Cauliflower, riced
1/4 cup Daikon radish, riced	1 large Chicken Breast, boneless

Roast the butternut squash in a 400 degree oven for about 15 to 20 minutes until it is fork tender. Let cool, then cut into cubes. Cut chicken into cubes.

Use either frozen cauliflower or fresh cauliflower to make cauli-rice. Cook for about two minutes in the microwave then put in a food processor. Clean, peel and cut the daikon into large cubes and add them to the food processor. Pulse until the vegetables are the size of rice.

Add 1 tablespoon of olive oil to a medium-sized skillet. When hot, add the cauliflower and daikon mixture and stir it around to slightly brown it. Add 1/2 cup water and mix well. Reduce heat to medium and cover. Allow the cauli-rice to cook until it is done, adding a little water if needed, about 20 minutes.

Heat olive oil in a large skillet or pan over medium heat. Add chicken and cook until it turns white. Remove to a bowl. Add a little more olive oil, then add onion and ginger garlic paste and sauté until it is soft, about 5 minutes. Add chicken broth and coconut milk, then cut curry paste square into smaller pieces and add to the liquid, stirring until the pieces melt and are mixed in together. Turn heat to a simmer.

Add chicken and let cook about 10 minutes, then add butternut squash and lime juice. Simmer until the chicken is completely cooked.

Serve with 1/2 of cauli-rice and a salad.

Nutrition Info per serving (includes cauli-rice)
Calories: 202 Fat: 8.1g Net Carbs:12.2g Protein: 15.7g

Rene Averett

Salmon Cakes With Dill Sauce

These salmon cakes are so good that I have to fight the cats off when I make them. They have their own version with fewer spices and no breading, but that doesn't mean that they don't want bites of mine as well. This would probably work just as well with crab or tuna, but I haven't gotten past the salmon to try them. (Photo on page 84.)

1/2 tablespoon Extra-Virgin Olive Oil, divided
1/4 cup Onion, finely chopped
1/2 cup Celery, finely diced
1 tablespoons chopped Parsley, fresh
3/4 cup cooked Salmon, flaked
1 large Egg, lightly beaten
1 tablespoon Mayonnaise
1 teaspoon Dijon Mustard
1/4 teaspoon Old Bay Spice or other seafood spice
1/2 cup Flax Bread Rolls (about 1 roll), processed to crumbs
1/4 teaspoon freshly ground Pepper

Prepare the Dill Sauce on page 83 and refrigerate until ready to use.

Preheat oven to 450°F. Coat a baking sheet with cooking spray.

Heat half the oil in a small skillet over medium-high heat. Add onion and celery; cook, stirring, until softened, about 3 minutes. Stir in parsley; remove from the heat.

In a medium bowl, flake salmon apart with a fork. Remove any bones and skin. Add egg, mayonnaise, and mustard and mix well. Add the onion mixture, breadcrumbs and seasonings and mix. Shape the mixture into 4 patties, about 2 1/2 inches wide.

Heat remaining oil in the pan over medium heat. Add patties and cook until the undersides are golden, 2 to 3 minutes. Using a wide spatula, turn them over onto the prepared baking sheet.

Bake the salmon cakes until golden on top and heated through, 15 to 20 minutes. Serve cakes with Dill Sauce and lemon wedges

Makes 2 servings

Nutrition Info per serving
  Calories: 228 Fat: 11.4g Net Carbs: 2.7g Protein: 25.6g

Creamy Dill Sauce

1/4 cup Mayonnaise
1 tablespoons Sour Cream
1 Green Onion (scallions), thinly sliced
1/2 tablespoon Lemon Juice
1/2 tablespoon finely chopped fresh Dill*
Freshly ground Black Pepper, to taste

Combine mayonnaise, yogurt, scallions, lemon juice, dill (or parsley) and pepper in a small bowl and mix well.

*You can use dried dill if fresh isn't available. Or you can substitute parsley, but then it isn't a dill sauce.

Nutrition Info per serving:
Calories: 209.3 g Fat: 22.8 g Net Carbs: 1.0 g Protein: 0.5 g

Feline Version

1 egg
1/2 can of Salmon or Tuna
2 tablespoons Flour
2 tablespoons Shredded or Grated Cheddar Cheese
Canned Shrimp to garnish, if desired
1 slice Bacon, cooked, broken into pieces to garnish

Preheat oven to 350°F. Break up salmon or tuna in a medium bowl and remove any bones. Lightly beat egg in a separate bowl, then combine with tuna. Add in flour and cheese. Stir to combine. Scoop batter into cupcake tin or silicone cups. Bake for 15 minutes. Cool, garnish and serve. Makes two or three small cakes.

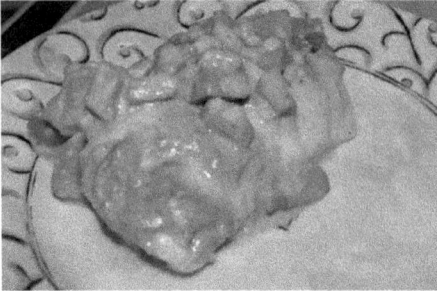

Peanut Curried Whitefish—pg 78

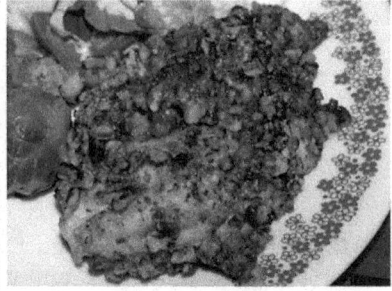

Pecan Crusted Chicken—pg 79

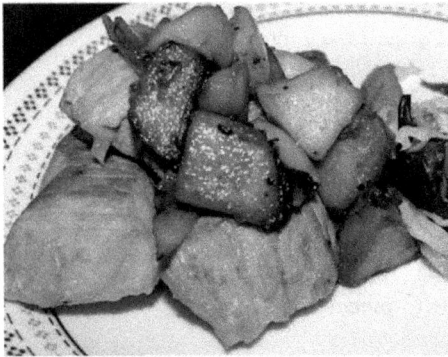

Pork, Butternut & Apple Sauté —pg 80

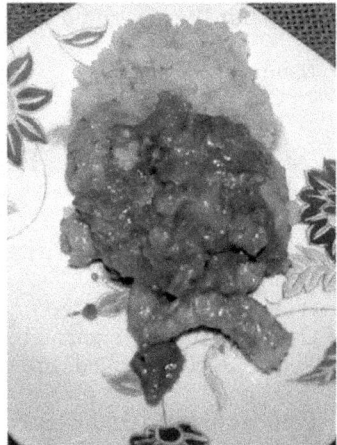

Pumpkin Shrimp Curry
with Cauli-rice—pg 81

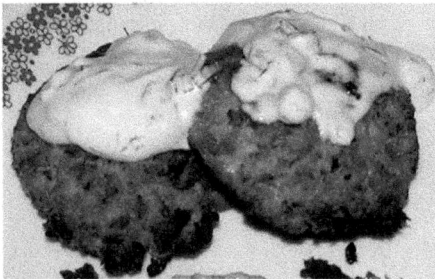

Salmon Cakes with Dill Sauce   pg 82

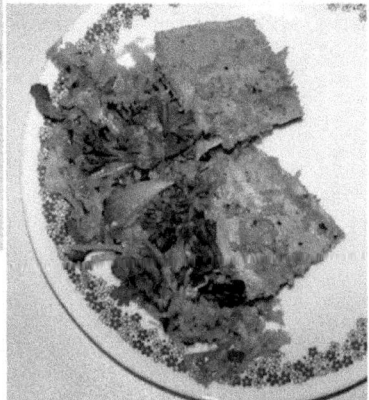

Irish Style Salmon with
Bacon & Cabbage —Pg 86

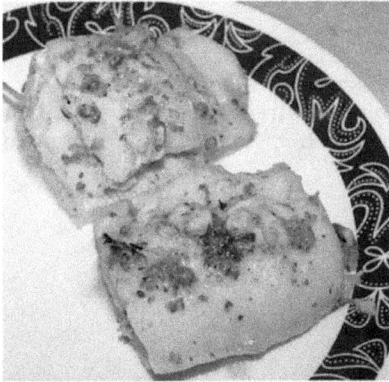

Crab Stuffed Cod—pg 88

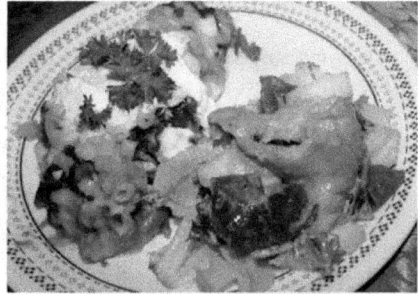

Salsa Chicken—pg 87

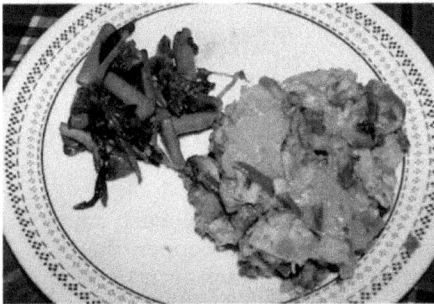

Quick Poached Whitefish—pg 89

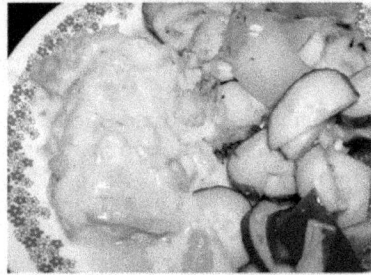

Scalloped Chicken & Turnips—pg 90

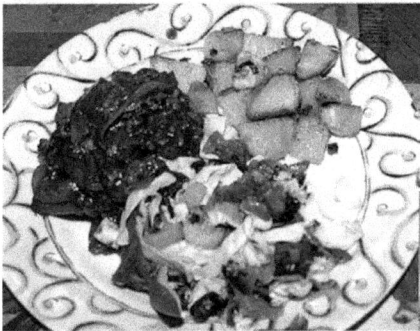

Chile Verde—pg 92

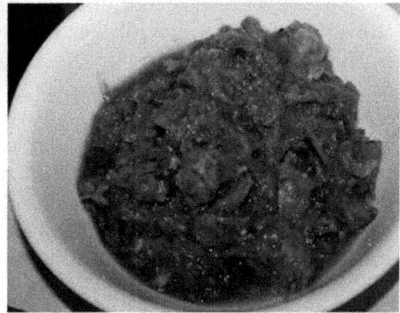

Simple Salisbury Steak—pg 91

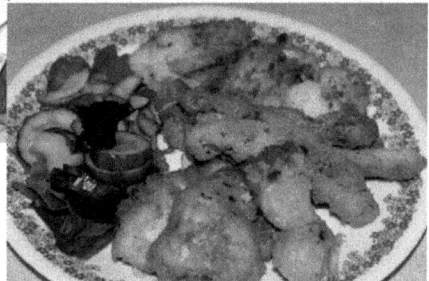

Tempura Cod & Vegetables—pg 93

Irish Style Salmon With Bacon and Cabbage

A variation on an Irish country dish, this combines the satisfying taste of braised shredded cabbage with bacon and a lightly seasoned salmon fillet. Simply delicious! If you can't find Irish bacon, use thick sliced bacon or Montana Cottage Bacon, which is similar. (Photo on page 84.)

1/4 head Savoy Cabbage, shredded
1/4 cup Onions, sliced
1 tablespoon Butter
1 tablespoons Red Wine
1/2 teaspoon Peppercorns
1/2 cup Chicken Stock
1 1/2 tablespoons Butter
2 Salmon Filets
4 slices Irish-style Bacon
1 tablespoon fresh Parsley

Cook the bacon in a large pan until done, but not crisp. Set on a paper towel to cool. Pour off all but 1 tablespoon of bacon oil. If you don't have enough, add butter to the pan. Add the onions and sauté until they are just tender.

Heat a non-stick skillet and add a little olive oil. Brush each side of the salmon with olive oil, season with a bit of salt and pepper, then put in the skillet to cook. Sear the salmon on one side, then turn to the other and sear it.

Break the bacon into smaller pieces and add it with the cabbage to onions and stir. Add the chicken stock. Cover with a tight fitting lid and continue to cook for 10 minutes, stirring occasionally. Add the salmon and cook until the salmon is cooked all the way though, about another 5 minutes. Serve on plates and sprinkle with fresh parsley.

Serves 2.

Nutrition Info per serving (3 oz. salmon)
  Calories: 286.3 Fat 18.6 g: Net Carbs:3.7 g Protein: 21.8 g

Salsa Chicken

This chicken recipe is easy to make and brings a lot of flavor to the table. The Mexican cheese is fresh tasting, milder than most cheeses, but if you can't find it, you can use a Jack Cheese instead. A nice thing about the Mexican cheese is that most of them are 0 carbohydrates. (Photo on page 85.)

    2 large Chicken Breast halves
    1 tablespoon Butter, melted
    3 teaspoons Taco Seasoning
    1/2 cup Mild or Medium Salsa*
    1/2 cup Cheddar Jack Cheese, shredded
    2 tablespoons Sour Cream
    2 tablespoons Green Onions, chopped
    2 tablespoons Queso Fresco or Asadero, crumbled

Heat oven to 375 degrees (F.).

Dip chicken breasts in butter, then sprinkle taco seasoning on top, pressing it into chicken. Place in an ungreased 8 inch square glass baking dish. Spoon salsa over the chicken.

Bake 30 minutes until the chicken is fork tender and juices run clear. Sprinkle cheeses over the chicken and bake another 5 minutes until the cheese is melted. Top with sour cream and green onions.

Great with Avocado Cucumber salad and Green Cauli-rice.

*Check the carb count on your salsa. They vary a bit, ranging from 1 net carb to 4 or 5 nc per 2 tablespoons. I used Glen Muir Black Bean and Corn Salsa that came in at a little less than 2 nc per 2 tablespoons, which is surprising for a salsa with beans and corn in it, although there isn't a lot of either. Each chicken breast or piece will use about 2 or 3 tablespoons to cover it.

Serves 2.

Nutrition Info per serving:
  Calories: 170.5 Fat: 10.6 g Net Carbs: 6.1 g Protein: 14.3 g

Crab Stuffed Cod

This is an elegant dish, but it isn't difficult to make. You will need low carb bread crumbs, so refer to the savory muffin recipe to make a bread that you can use for the crumbs. Alternately, use Progresso Italian style Bread Crumbs or a similar option, just look for the lowest carb count on the packaging. You are only using 2 tablespoons, so it will add about 2.3 net carbs per serving. (Photo on page 85.)

4 ounces Crab Meat
1 tablespoon Butter, melted
1 tablespoon Mayonnaise
2 tablespoons low carb Bread Crumbs
1 tablespoon Parmesan Cheese
1/4 teaspoon dried Parsley
1/8 teaspoon Lemon Juice
1/8 teaspoon Garlic Pepper

1/2 pound Cod, about 1 inch thick
1/4 cup Chicken Broth or bullion
1/2 teaspoon Lemon Juice
1 tablespoon Butter, melted
1/2 teaspoon Parsley
1 tablespoon Heavy Cream

Preheat oven to 350 degrees (F.)

Prepare the crab stuffing. Mix the butter, mayonnaise, Parmesan cheese, bread crumbs, parsley, lemon juice and garlic pepper together. Stir in the crab and set aside.

Divide the cod into two pieces. Cut a pocket into the long side of the fish and cut almost through. Spoon 1/2 the crab filling into each cod filet. Secure with a toothpick.

Mix the chicken broth, melted butter, lemon juice, parsley and heavy cream together, then pour into the bottom of a small baking pan. Put the two stuffed cod pieces into the pan. Drizzle with olive oil and sprinkle lightly with additional bread crumbs if desired.

Bake for 30 to 35 minutes until the cod is completely done and the sauce is bubbly. Serve on plate, spooning the sauce over the top.

Makes 2 servings.

Nutrition Info per serving
  Calories: 369 Fat: 21.8 g Net Carbs: 1.7g Protein: 39.5 g

Quick Poached White Fish

When I first wanted to do a poached fish, I thought it would be a simple process, but the recipes all seemed more complicated than I wanted. I finally hit on this one, which is easy and quick to do. (Photo on page 85.)

2 White Fish filets, about 1/2" thick
1/4 cup Onions, sliced
1 tablespoon Low Carb Flour
1 tablespoon Butter
1/2 cup Heavy Whipping Cream
1/4 cup White Wine
1 tablespoon Lemon Juice

Preheat the oven to 350 degrees F.

Butter a baking dish that can go from stove to oven. I used a 1 quart cast iron or cast aluminum pot with a lid. Layer the sliced onions on the bottom, then put the fish fillets on top and dot with butter. I also sprinkled about a tablespoon of dried chives on top. Cover the fish with the white wine and water. Bring to a simmer. Cover with a lid or heavy aluminum foil and cook in the oven for 8 to 10 minutes.

Remove the fish fillets to a plate or tin and cover with foil to keep warm while you prepare the sauce. If the fish isn't quite done, it will continue to cook while it rests.

Make the sauce in the pan you baked the fish in. Mix flour and butter together to make a paste, put in a little of the juice and mix until it is smooth, adding more liquid as needed until you can easily add it to the juices in the pan. Add cream, then cook and stir until the sauce thickens. (If it won't thicken, use a little low carb thickener like Thick It Up, or guar gum powder or a teaspoon of cornstarch.)

Spoon the sauce over the fish and serve. Makes two servings (and a bite or two for the cat or dog).

Nutrition Info:
Calories: 287 Fat: 18.3 g Net Carbs: 2.9 g Protein: 22.3 g

Scalloped Chicken & Turnips

This is an adaptation of a recipe for Chicken and Scalloped potatoes that was made with a mix. Tossing out the potatoes, I've replaced them with a combination of turnips, cauliflower and Daikon radish. For a thickener, I've used my secret ingredient, pumpkin puree. This dish just might become your new favorite. (Photo on page 85.)

1 large Turnip, sliced thinly
1/4 cup fresh Cauliflower, sliced thinly
1/2 cup Heavy Cream
1 cup cubed cooked Chicken
2 tablespoon Pumpkin Puree
1/2 cup frozen Green Beans
1/4 cup sliced Mushrooms
1 tablespoon Butter
1/4 cup low carb Bread Crumbs
2 tablespoons Butter, melted
1 tablespoon chopped fresh Parsley
1 tablespoon chopped Chives

Preheat oven to 450 degrees (F)

Slice the turnips, cauliflower and radish thinly, then put into a microwavable bowl. Cook in microwave for three minutes with a cover over the bowl. Put vegetables into a one quart casserole dish with the chicken, green beans, pumpkin and mushrooms. Stir to mix well. Add nutmeg to the heavy cream and mix, then pour over the chicken and vegetables mix. Cut 1 tablespoon butter over the top. Bake for 25 minutes.

Remove the casserole from the oven and stir the mixture. Return to the oven and bake another 10 minutes.

Mix low carb bread crumbs with melted butter, poultry seasoning and fresh parsley. Remove the casserole again and top with the bread crumb mixture, distributing it evenly around the dish. Put back in the oven for another 5 minutes.

Serves 4.

Nutrition Info:
Calories: 332 Fat: 26.0 g Net Carbs: 4.5 g Protein: 17.8 g

Simple Salisbury Steak

This is a simple, satisfying skillet dish to make for two people using hamburger patties for the chopped steak in the recipe . A low carb sauce compliments the meat with onions and mushrooms in a wine sauce.

2 pre-made Hamburger or Ground Steak Patties
1/4 cup sliced Onions
1/4 cup sliced Mushrooms
1 tablespoon Beef Bouillon paste (Better Than Bouillon)
1 oz. Red Wine
1 teaspoon Worcestershire Sauce
1 tablespoon minced Garlic
1/4 teaspoon Sage
1 tablespoon Butter
Salt and Pepper to taste

Thaw the patties, then sprinkle salt, pepper and sage into the beef and press it into two patties about 1/2 inch thick.

In a skillet big enough for both patties, melt the butter, then add the garlic and onions. Sauté over medium heat until the garlic is fragrant, then add the mushrooms and cook a few minutes longer Remove the vegetables to a plate. Add the beef patties to the skillet and brown on one side, then flip to the other to brown that side also. Lower the heat to a simmer and cover.

Mix the bullion into the wine until it is smoothed into it, then add to the skillet. It will absorb the meat juices and bits of flavor in the skillet. Continue to cook for about 10 minutes until the meat is completely cooked and the sauce begins to thicken. Add the onions and mushrooms back to the pan and cook a few minutes more to heat them.

Serve with a cauliflower-turnip or kohlrabi mash and a freshly sautéed pan of shaved Brussels sprouts or broccoli.

Nutrition Info per serving:
Calories: 251 Fat: 14.1 g Net Carbs: 3.1 g Protein: 25.1 g

Pork Chile Verde

Chile Verde has been a staple in my life from childhood on. It is basically a green chile stew. In its purest form, it doesn't have red tomatoes in it, so I am always suspect when a Mexican restaurant serves me the dish with red stuff in it. This makes a Texas authentic version of the dish. (Photo on page 85.)

1 1/3 lbs Pork Butt or Shoulder,	1/2 teaspoon Salt
2 tablespoons Olive Oil	1/2 cup Onions, chopped
1/3 teaspoon ground Black Pepper	1 garlic Cloves, minced
2 tablespoons chopped Green Chiles	1 cup Tomatillos, chopped
1 tablespoon diced Jalapeno Pepper	1 teaspoon dried Oregano
2 tablespoons Coconut Flour	1 teaspoon ground Cumin
2 tablespoons Cilantro, chopped	1 cup Chicken Stock
1 1/2 teaspoons ground Coriander	

Trim the pork and cut into 1 inch cubes. Season with salt and pepper, then coat in coconut flour. In a heavy pot, heat oil over medium high heat and brown the pork cubes in batches. Turn to make sure all sides are browned. Remove pork from the pot with a slotted spoon and put in a bowl. Repeat with each batch.

Pour off excess fat, then add peppers and onions to the skillet and cook over medium heat, stirring now and then until they are tender, about five minutes. Add the canned chiles and garlic and cook a few more minutes.

Add the pork cubes, tomatillos, dried herbs and chopped cilantro, cover with chicken stock and bring to a boil then reduce to a simmer. With a wooden spoon, break tomatillos into smaller pieces as the stew cooks . Cook uncovered for 2-3 hours until the pork is fork tender.

Adjust the seasoning to taste with salt and pepper. Makes 4 servings.

Nutrition Info per serving:
  Calories: 603 Fat: 51.5 g Net Carbs: 6.9 g Protein: 38.9 g

Tempura Cod and Vegetables

The temptation of this Asian dish is too much to pass up sometimes, so this lower carb'd version may just fill the bill when you get a craving for it. If you can't find kohlrabi at your market, then try turnips or celery root as a substitute. (Photo on page 85.)

2 4 oz pieces of Cod, cut into three chunks each
1/2 cup Zucchini, cut into large cubes
1/2 cup Kohlrabi, sliced into 1/4" slices
6 cleaned fresh Green Beans
1 recipe Tempura Batter (next page)

Wash fish off and cut into chunks. Cut all the vegetables into 1inch to 1 ½ inch chunks. Bring a pot of water to boil and parboil the cut vegetables for about three minutes to pre-cook them a bit. Drain, then dry off with a paper towel.

Mix the tempura batter. Add ice water until it has a thick, but not too thick consistency. It needs to stick to the food, but not make too thick a coating. When using coconut flour, it will absorb liquid, so it will use at least double and possibly three times as much water as the recipe calls for.

Pour oil to about 1 1/2 inch deep in a deep skillet (I use cast iron) and heat to 375 degrees, or until a bit of batter sizzles and browns quickly. Lower the heat slightly. Try to keep an even heat.

Dip about six vegetables in the tempura batter, then place gently in the oil to fry. It will take just a few minutes for them to brown on one side. Turn with a slotted spatula and brown on the other side. Remove to a paper towel covered plate to drain. Continue to cook vegetables, about six to a batch. You can keep the drained vegetables warm in a 225 degree oven on a baking tin. Fry the chunks of fish last. They will take about 3 to 5 minutes a side, depending on thickness. Check to be sure the fish is cooked all the way through.

Serve as soon as possible. You can sprinkle with rice vinegar or any favorite flavor of sauce you like. Left over vegetables and fish don't reheat very well, but you can put them on a baking sheet and warm them in the oven for about 10 minutes at 300 degrees.

Nutrition Info per serving without batter:
Calories: 140.4 Fat: 0.1g Net Carbs: 2.5 g Protein: 26.4 g

Note: The amount of food you can dip in one cup of batter will vary depending on the size of the pieces. So basically, divide the total carbs in the Tempura recipe by the number of pieces of fish and vegetables in each serving and add it to the total above. On average, it should be about 7 net carbs per serving.

Tempura Batter

Use this recipe for tempura batter for the Cod and Vegetables. You can use it with any vegetables, shrimp, chicken and pork. Be creative!

1/4 cup Low Carb Baking Mix
1/4 cup Coconut Flour
1/2 teaspoon Baking Powder
1/2 teaspoon Salt
1 Egg
1/3 cup Ice Cold Water
Oil for deep frying

Sift the dry ingredients together and set aside. In a medium bowl, beat the egg slightly and mix with the ice water. Stir in the dry ingredients until mixed. The batter will be slightly lumpy.

Dip meat, fish or vegetables into the batter. Heat oil to 375 degrees or until it sizzles. Fry the food in small batches, about six at a time until golden brown, turn and brown the other side.

Remove to a paper towel to drain, then put on a plate or tin in a warm oven to keep hot.

Alternate Version:

If you have low carb pancake batter, such as New Hope Mills Pancake Mix, you can mix up 1 cup of batter and use it as a tempura batter.

Nutrition Info for batter recipe:
Calories: 568.5 Fat: 55.87 g Net Carbs: 8.7 g Protein: 10.8 g

Super Sides

Great side dishes compliment your dinners and lunches. These are not your ordinary vegetables, although some you do use commonly may be playing a different role. In low carb eating, you want to avoid fruits and vegetables that are high in sugars and starches, which add the carbohydrates to the meal. These dishes use vegetables such as turnips, kohlrabi, celery root, daikon radish and cauliflower to substitute for potatoes, rice and pasta. This gives you fewer carbs in your meal and leaves room for the wonderful desserts, which are coming up in the next chapter.

Avocado Cucumber Salad	96
E-Z Vegetable Fries	96
Broccoli Salad	97
Asparagus & Leek Cauli-Risotto	98
Grandma's Tex-Mex Spanish Cauli-rice	99
Green Cauli Rice	100
Home-style Veggies O'Brien	101
Mexicali Esparragus con el Nabo	104
Orange & Pecan Roasted Brussels Sprouts	105
Smashed Turnips with Cauliflower & Cheddar	106
Springtime Coleslaw	107
Turnip & Cauliflower Gratin	108
Zucchini, Spinach & Bacon Fritters	109

Avocado Cucumber Salad

This lovely salad brings in the southwest flavors beautifully and is so colorful. Try it with your favorite Mexican dish. (Pictured on page 102.)

1/2 Avocado, diced
1/2 Cucumber, peeled and diced
1/4 cup Red Onion, diced
1/2 cup Tomato, diced
1 tablespoon fresh Cilantro, chopped
1 teaspoon Lemon or Lime juice
2 tablespoons Mayonnaise
1/2 teaspoon Cayenne Pepper
1/2 teaspoon Cumin
2 tablespoons Queso Fresco or Asadero (optional)

Mix lemon or lime juice, mayonnaise, cayenne pepper and cumin together.

In a medium bowl, combine avocado, cucumber, red onion and tomato. Stir in the dressing and cilantro then turn over several times with a spoon to mix it in well. Cover bowl with a plastic wrap and chill for 2 hours before serving. Sprinkle with a little Queso Fresco or Asadero on top when serving, if you wish.

Makes 2 servings.

Nutrition Info per serving:
  Calories: 186.6 Fat: 6.2 g Net Carbs: 3.7 g Protein: 3.1 g

E-Z Vegetable Fries

Quick and easy veggie fries that rival potatoes. (Pictured on cover)

2/3 cup Celery Root, Kohlrabi or Turnips, sliced into planks
Olive Oil or Coconut Oil to coat pan about ¼ inch deep
Seasoning Salt

Boil a pan of water and par boil the root vegetable for about three minutes. Put on paper towel to dry.
Heat the oil in a small skillet until it is sizzling hot. Turn to medium high heat. Fry the vegetables, a few at a time until lightly browned on both sides. Put on a paper towel to drain. Let the fries cool for a bit, then fry them a second time until golden brown. Drain, season and serve.
Makes 2 servings

Nutrition Info per serving:
  Calories: 41 Fat: 2.4 g Net Carbs: 3.8 g Protein: 0.7 g

Broccoli Salad

This is the summer picnic standby salad, the alternate to potato salad and it's so refreshing. It can also be made low carb with just a few little changes. The best part is that practically no one will notice. (Pictured on page 102.)

1 cup Broccoli, chopped
1/4 cup Red Onions, chopped
1/8 cup Sunflower Seeds, hulled
1/2 cup Mayonnaise
3 tablespoons Bacon Pieces
1 tablespoons Lemon Juice
1 1/2 tablespoons Sugar Substitute
3 tablespoons Craisins Reduced Sugar
1/4 cup Cheddar Cheese, grated (optional)
Pinch of salt

Chop Broccoli into bite-sized or smaller pieces. I use a food processor, so the pieces get very small, but you can use larger pieces if you prefer. Chop onions to very small pieces.

In a large mixing bowl, add the broccoli, onions, crasins, bacon and sunflower seeds. In a small bowl, mix the mayonnaise, lemon juice and sugar substitute together to make the sauce. Add a bit of salt. Pour the mayonnaise dressing over the broccoli and mix it well. If you like, add the grated cheese and mix it in or just put it on top until served.

Makes 4 servings

Nutrition Info per serving:
Calories: 298 Fat: 27.0 g Net Carbs: 6.7 g Protein: 6.1 g

Asparagus & Leek Cauli-Risotto

Absolutely delicious and a very beautiful dish. Try it when asparagus is in season. (Pictured on page 102.)

1 cup Cauliflower, raw
1/2 cup Daikon Radish
1/2 cup Asparagus, fresh
1/4 cup Mushrooms, fresh
1/2 cup Leeks, slices (bottom only)
1/2 cup Chicken Broth or Bouillon,
1/4 teaspoon Salt
1/4 teaspoon Lemon Pepper seasoning
1/4 cup White Wine
1 cloves of Garlic
1/2 tablespoon Butter
3 tablespoons Parmesan cheese

Cut cauliflower into pieces and microwave for about 5 minutes to partially cook. If using frozen cauliflower, microwave about 2 minutes to defrost. Peel the daikon and cut into cubes. Put cauliflower and daikon in food processor and pulse until the pieces are about the size of rice. Set aside.

Cut asparagus into one inch segments on a diagonal and microwave in a bowl for about 30 seconds to just slightly steam. Cut or break mushrooms into pieces. Finely chop two cloves of garlic. Slice leek into thin slices.

Melt butter in a deep skillet, brown garlic until just golden brown. Add leeks, then add the cauliflower and daikon mixture and stir together in the skillet. Add one cup of water and stir it around. Cook on high heat until it boils, then reduce the heat to a simmer. Add 1/2 cup of bouillon or chicken broth and stir in. Cook until the liquid is absorbed, stirring every five or so minutes. When almost all the liquid is gone, add white wine, asparagus, mushrooms and seasonings.

Cook over low heat until the liquid is almost gone and the dish is just moist. Sprinkle on cheese and serve.

Makes 2 servings

Nutrition Info per serving:
  Calories: 124 Fat: 5.7 g Net Carbs: 6.4 g Protein: 5.8 g

Grandma's Tex-Mex Spanish Cauli-rice

My grandmother made the best Tex-Mex Spanish rice ever, so I knew I had to recreate it in a low carb version. While cauliflower isn't rice, it does an admirable job subbing for it with this recipe. The flavors take over the dish and what's surprising is how much this dish tastes like Spanish rice. In fact, I like it better. If you don't have a food processor, you can also grate the cauliflower. (Pictured on page 102.)

1 cup Cauliflower, fresh or frozen
1/2 cup canned Diced Tomatoes
2 tablespoons Sweet Peppers, thinly sliced or chopped
2 tablespoons Onions, chopped
1 teaspoon Chicken Bouillon paste
1/4 cup Water
1/2 teaspoon minced Garlic
1/2 teaspoon Chili powder
1/2 teaspoon Seasoning Salt
1 teaspoon Olive Oil or Butter

Parboil the cauliflower for 3 minutes, then drain. Put in a food processor and pulse until the cauliflower is the size of rice.

In a medium skillet, sauté garlic and onion in olive oil or butter over medium heat. Add canned tomatoes, 1/4 cup of water and cauliflower and stir well. Add the chopped peppers and seasoning, then cover the pan and reduce the heat to a simmer. Let cook, stirring a couple of times, until the liquid is reduced and the cauliflower is tender, between 25 and 30 minutes.

Serves 2.

Nutrition info per serving:
Calories: 50.4 Fat: 2.1 Net Carbs: 4.7g Protein: 1.8 g

Green Cauli Rice

For variety, this version of cauli-rice goes well with Mexican food or Asian food. It gets its green from the added vegetables and the sauce made with green chili salsa. It is a lovely side dish with a mildly spicy flavor.

1 cup Cauliflower pieces
1/4 cup Daikon Radish
1/2 teaspoon Chicken Bullion
1/4 cup Bell Pepper, sliced
1/4 cup Anaheim Pepper, sliced
1 cup Zucchini
1/4 cup sliced Green Onions
1/4 cup Green Chili Salsa or 1/4 cup Green Enchilada Sauce
1/2 teaspoon Garlic Powder
1/2 teaspoon Seasoning Salt
1/4 teaspoon Black Pepper, ground
1 tablespoon Butter
1/2 cup Water

Put the cauliflower, daikon, peppers, onions and zucchini in a food processor and pulse until the vegetables are the size of large grains of rice.

In a medium skillet, melt the butter over medium high heat, then add the riced vegetables. Add the seasonings, bullion and water. Bring to a boil, then lower heat to simmer. Cover and cook for about 20 minutes, checking a couple of times to make sure all the liquid hasn't been cooked out. Add the salsa or sauce and stir. Add a little more water if needed, then cook another 5 to 10 minutes until the vegetables resemble fluffy rice. You want it moist, but not too wet.

Serves 2.

Nutrition info per serving:
Calories:90.9 Fat:6.2 g Net Carbs: 3.7 g Protein: 3.1 g

Home-style Veggies O'Brien

A tasty mix of several root vegetables with cauliflower to make a dish similar to Potatoes O'Brien, without the high carbs! Don't like daikon? Just sub in more kohlrabi or turnip, Don't like turnip or cauliflower? Sub in whichever of the root vegetables you like. (Pictured on page 102.)

Don't know what kohlrabi is? Look for the green 3" or more globe vegetable that's about the color of broccoli and has many stems, possibly with leaves, coming up from the globe. The flavor is similar to the broccoli stem and is delicately-flavored without being overwhelming.

1/4 cup Cauliflower, cut into pieces
1/4 cup Kohlrabi, cut into 1/4" cubes
1/4 cup Turnips, cut into 1/4" cubes
1/4 cup Daikon Radish, cut into 1/4" cubes
1/4 cup Onions, chopped
2 tablespoons Sweet Peppers, sliced
1/2 tablespoon Olive Oil or Bacon Fat
1/2 teaspoon Seasoning Salt or Garlic Pepper Seasoning

Put cauliflower, kohlrabi, turnips and daikon in a pot, cover with water and boil for about 15 minutes. Drain. In a skillet, heat olive oil, add onions and peppers and stir fry until tender. Add vegetables and stir together. Cook, stirring often, until veggies are lightly browned. Add seasoning and serve.

Makes two 1/2 cup servings.

Nutrition info per serving:
Calories: 35.2 Fat: 0.2 g Net Carbs:3.4 g Protein: 1.0 g

Note: You can cook up the vegetables ahead of time and store in the refrigerator in a plastic bag for about a week or freeze to store longer. Just pull them out when you're ready to make your hash browns.

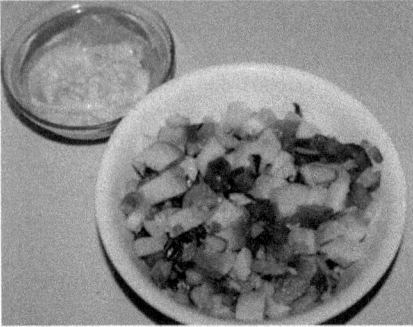

Avocado Cucumber Salad—pg 96

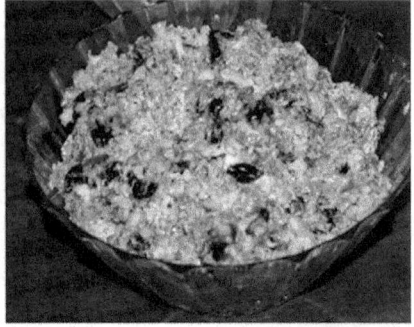

Broccoli Salad—pg 97

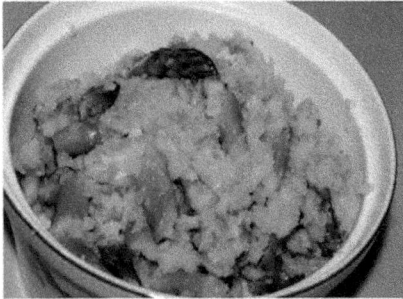

Asparagus Leek Risotto—pg 98

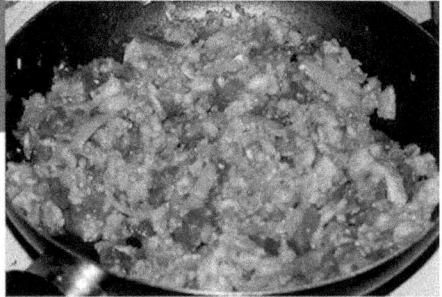

Grandma's Tex-Mex Spanish
Cauli-rice—pg 99

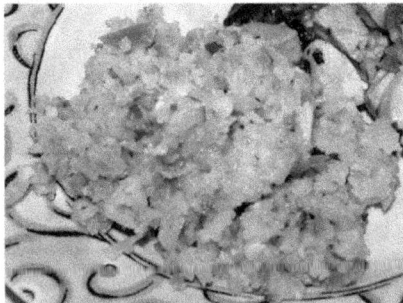

Green Cauli-rice—pg 100

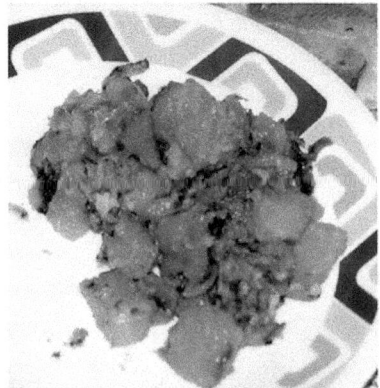

Home-style Veggies O'Brien—pg 101

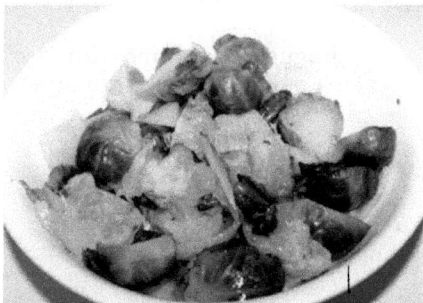

Orange & Pecan Roasted Brussels Sprouts—pg 105

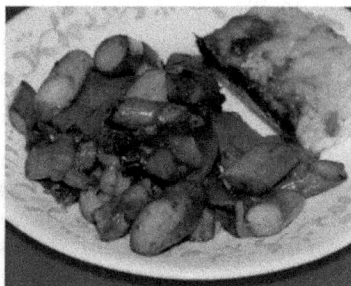

Mexicali Esparragus—pg 104

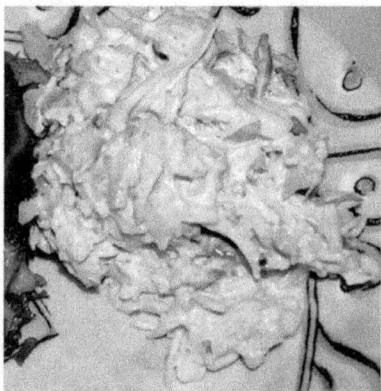

Smashed Turnips and Cauliflower
with Cheese—pg 106

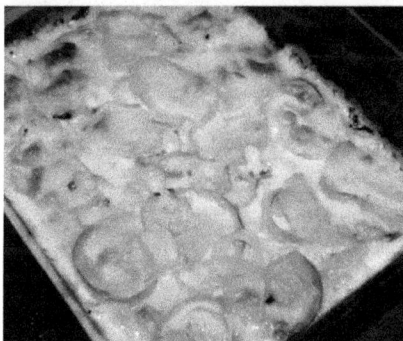

Springtime Coleslaw—pg 107

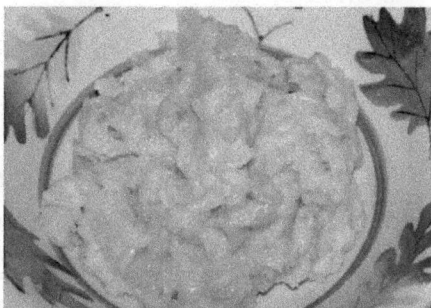

Zucchini, Bacon & Turnip Fritters—pg 109

Turnip & Cauliflower Gratin—pg 108

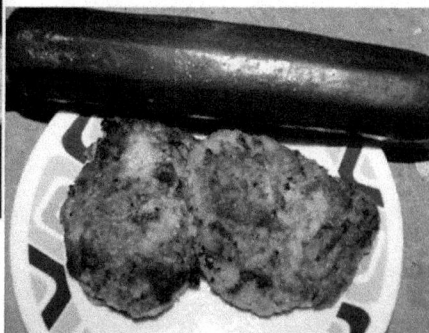

Mexicali Esparragus con el Nabo

This is a tasty Mexican-style dish of asparagus and turnips with Pico de Gallo added to spice the dish. The Spanish name just gives it a little flair. (Pictured on page 103.)

You can buy Pico de Gallo in many grocery stores, but if you can't find it, chop 1/2 medium tomato, 1/4 of a medium onion, 1/2 small jalapeno pepper, seeds removed, and a bit of fresh garlic and combine together. Add about one tablespoon of chopped cilantro.

4 large Asparagus Spears
1/2 medium Turnip (about ½ cup)
2 Green Onions
1/8 cup Celery Hearts and Leaves
1 tablespoon minced Garlic
1/4 cup Pico de Gallo
1/2 teaspoon Sugar Substitute
1/2 teaspoon Mrs Dash Tomato, Basil and Garlic powder
1/2 tablespoon Olive Oil

Wash and trim asparagus, then cut into 1 inch pieces.

Peel turnip and cut into thin slices. Put turnip in a microwavable dish, add 1/4 cup water and sugar substitute. Microwave for 2 minutes, then drain. If you prefer, bring water to boil in a pot and parboil the turnip for 3 minutes rather than microwaving.

Chop green onions and celery hearts and leaves.

In a medium skillet, heat olive oil and add garlic, then onions and celery. Stir until slightly brown, then add the turnips. Cook for about 5 minutes until turnips are just browning. Add asparagus and continue to stir-cook the vegetables. When the asparagus are crisp-tender, add the Pico de Gallo and stir-cook about another 2 to 3 minutes.

Serves 2.

Nutrition Info per serving:
Calories 62 Fat: 4.0 g Net Carbs: 4.7 g Protein: 1.6 g

Orange & Pecan Roasted Brussels Sprouts

This is a recipe suggestion from my local grocery store that is really not in need of much adapting to low carb at all since it already is. However, like a certain TV chef or two, I do add my own spin on it by adding a citrus taste to it. (Pictured on page 103.)

1 cup Brussels Sprouts, trimmed and sliced
1/2 tablespoon Olive Oil
1/4 teaspoon Salt
1/4 teaspoon freshly ground Pepper
1/3 Onion, thinly sliced
1/4 cup chopped Oranges
1/2 teaspoon Lemon Juice
1/4 teaspoon Thyme
2 tablespoons Pecans or Walnuts, broken into pieces

Preheat oven to 400 degrees (F.) Prepare a baking sheet with a sheet of foil sprayed with cooking spray.

Cut Brussels sprouts in half and place in medium mixing bowl. Toss in olive oil, salt, freshly ground pepper, orange pieces and lemon juice.

Spread the vegetable mix on the prepared baking sheet and top with onion slices and a few sprinkles of thyme. Roast for 10 minutes. Add coarsely chopped nuts and roast another 10 minutes, stirring every a couple of times until they nuts are toasted and the sprouts are done. If the sprouts get a bit charred, that is okay, but don't burn the nuts.

Makes two servings.

Nutrition info per serving:
Calories: 124 Fat: 9.2 g Net Carbs: 7.0 g Protein: 2.7 g

Smashed Turnips with Cauliflower & Cheddar

You cannot believe how wonderful the combination of turnips and cauliflower with cheddar cheese tastes. Potatoes? Who needs potatoes? These are great! (Pictured on page 103.)

1 1/2 medium Turnips, cubed (1 medium, 1 small)
1 tablespoon Heavy Cream
1 tablespoon Butter
1/4 cup sharp Cheddar Cheese, shredded or cubed
Salt and Pepper to taste
1/4 teaspoon Paprika
1/2 teaspoon Sugar Substitute
1/4 cup Bacon pieces (optional)
1 tablespoon Chives, chopped

In a small saucepan, add cubed turnips and enough water to cover. Bring to a boil, then reduce heat to medium high and cook until the vegetables are tender, about 15 to 20 minutes.

When fork tender, drain the water off, then either put in the food processor and pulse several times until the turnips are a chunky puree or put back in the pan and hand mash with a masher or fork until they are the consistency you like. Put the smashed turnips back in the pan, add the butter, sugar substitute and seasonings. Cook over low heat to get any excess water out and melt the butter. Add the cheese, and heavy cream and stir together until the cheese melts and is mixed in completely.

Turn off heat, stir in the chopped chives and bacon, if you are adding them.

Serves 2

Nutrition Info per servings (with optional bacon)
Calories: 234 Fat: 19g Net Carbs: 4.5g Protein: 11.3g

Springtime Coleslaw

Easy to make and totally refreshing, this coleslaw will brighten up any lunch or dinner and is great for summer picnics. (Pictured on page 103.)

1/4 cup Mayonnaise
1/4 tablespoons Sugar Substitute
1/4 tablespoon Brown Sugar Substitute
1/4 teaspoon ground Ginger
2 tablespoons chopped Pecans or Walnuts
1/4 cup Brussels Sprouts, shredded and chopped
2 medium Asparagus Spears, chopped
2 tablespoons crushed fresh Pineapple (not canned)
1/4 (16 ounce) package shredded Coleslaw Mix
1 tablespoon Heavy Cream

In a medium bowl, mix mayonnaise, sugars, ginger, nuts, pineapple and cream to make the dressing

Toss coleslaw mix, asparagus and Brussels sprouts with dressing to coat.

Chill at least 1 hour before serving.

Makes 2 servings

Nutrition Info per serving:
Calories: 248 Fat: 5.0 g Net Carbs: 2.9 g Protein: 1.7 g

Turnip & Cauliflower Gratin

The combination of turnips with cauliflower works beautifully to make a wonderfully satisfying gratin dish. If you don't like turnips, you can substitute kohlrabi or celery root for the turnips, or just use all cauliflower. (Pictured on page 103.)

1/2 cup Turnips, sliced thinly
1/2 cup Cauliflower, sliced thinly
1/4 cup Onion, sliced thinly
1/2 cup Heavy Whipping Cream,
1/4 teaspoon Cayenne Pepper
1/4 teaspoon Thyme, ground or 1 tablespoon fresh
1/4 teaspoon Salt
1 cloves Garlic, smashed
1 teaspoon Fresh Chives or 1/4 teaspoon dried Chives
1/3 cup Mozzarella Cheese or Parmesan Cheese, shredded
1 tablespoon Butter

Put the cream and seasonings, except chives, into a small saucepan and bring to a boil. Turn off the heat and taste to check the seasonings. Adjust, if needed. Let the mixture sit for 15 to 20 minutes.

Preheat oven to 375 degrees (F.) Lightly spray a small baking dish with cooking spray or butter the bottom and sides.

Peel turnips and boil them for 20 minutes. Cut into thin slices as evenly as possible. If you use a mandolin to cut, then cut the slices before cooking and only cook about 5 minutes to soften them. Drain. Cut 1/4 head of cauliflower into slices, put in a bowl and microwave for 4 minutes to partially cook. Cut a small onion into thin slices. You should have about 1/4 cup.

Layer 1/2 of the turnips on the bottom of the pan and dot with 1/2 tablespoon of butter. Remove the garlic from the sauce and spoon about 1/3 over the turnips. Sprinkle with 1/3 of the cheese. Layer the cauliflower and onions on top of the first layer, dot with butter and spoon 1/3 of the sauce over the top and sprinkle with 1/3 of the cheese.. Layer the rest of the turnips over the top layer, dot with the remaining butter, pour the rest of the sauce over the top, and sprinkle the remaining cheese on top. Sprinkle a little paprika over the top if you would like.

Cook at 375 degrees (F) for 35 minutes. Remove cover and bake another 15 minutes until golden brown.

Makes 2 servings

Nutrition Info per serving:
Calories: 195 Fat: 17.4 g Net Carbs: 4.2 g Protein: 5.1 g

Zucchini, Spinach & Bacon Fritters

These are so incredibly good that you'll want to make them again and again. They are a great side dish or wonderful for snacks. (Pictured on page 103.)

1 medium Zucchini, shredded
1 slice of Bacon, fried, bacon grease reserved
1/4 cup cut fresh Spinach
2 tablespoons shredded Parmesan Cheese
1 Egg
2 tablespoons Low Carb Flour or Almond or Coconut Flour
1/4 teaspoon Baking Powder
1/4 teaspoon ground Thyme
1/4 teaspoon Paprika
1/8 teaspoon dried Celeriac, crushed
1/8 teaspoon ground black Pepper and Garlic

Put shredded zucchini in a bowl and add 1/2 teaspoon sea salt. Let sit 10 minutes or more. Pour water off, then squeeze the zucchini to get additional water out of it. Blot with a paper towel to remove more water.

Put the zucchini in a quart plastic bag. Crumble the bacon and add to the bag. Cut the spinach into small pieces and add to the bag with the Parmesan cheese and the seasonings. Add the egg, close the bag and smush it around to mix the ingredients. Add the baking powder and flour and close the bag again and smush it until all the flour is mixed in and you have a moist pancake-like batter.

Heat a heavy skillet, such as a cast iron one, over medium heat and add about 1 tablespoon of the reserved bacon grease. If you don't have enough add a little olive oil. When the grease is hot, put a tablespoon of the batter on one side of the skillet and smooth it into a round or oval with the back of the spoon. Put another tablespoon on the opposite side. Cook for about four minutes and lift to see if it will flip easily. If it will, then flip the pancake over and cook another four minutes on the back side. Watch the heat with these or they will burn on the bottom.

Remove to a paper towel on a plate to drain. Repeat with the next batch. The recipe makes 4 fritters.

Serve with salad dressing or sour cream with chives or a Dill Sauce.

Nutrition info per fritter:
  Calories: 55.1 Fat:3.3 g Net Carbs: 1.7 g Protein: 3.9 g

Devine Desserts

A bit of sweetness is sometimes called for to top off a dinner meal. Just because you're living low carb doesn't mean you can't enjoy some enticing dessert options. These selections are all under 10 net carbs and some as low as 2 net carbs per serving. So, indulge a little.

Almond Tea Biscuits	112
Caramel Nut Cheesecake	113
Coconut Flour Flaugnarde	114
Cranberry Pumpkin Biscotti Cookies	115
Cranberry Peach Cobbler	116
Espresso Hazelnut Custard & Bourbon Sauce	119
Blueberry Dumplings	120
Peanut Butter Blossom Cookies	121
Peanut Butter Chocolate Cake	122
Raspberry Lemon Drop Tart	123
Sour Cream Lemon Cake	124
Cranberry Chocolate Pecan Pie Tarts	125
Pumpkin Cheese Mousse	126
Pumpkin Flan	127
Chocolate Mist Cheesecake	128

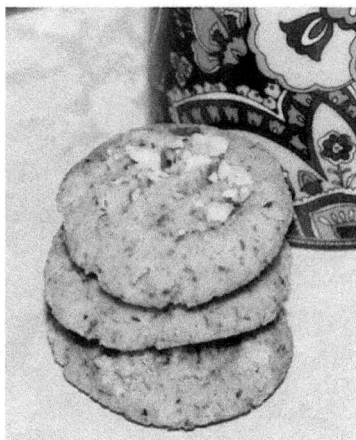

Almond Tea Biscuits—pg 112

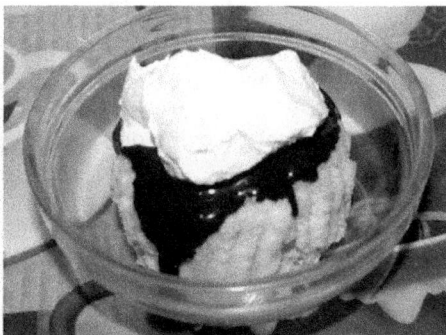

Caramel Nut Cheesecake—pg 113

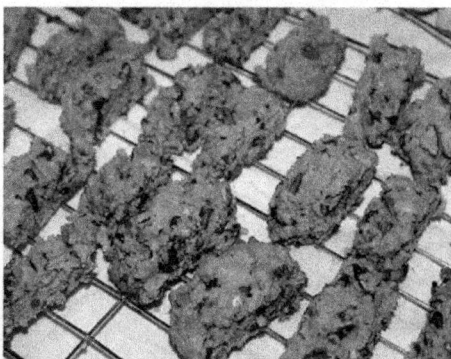

Cranberry Pumpkin Biscotti—pg 115

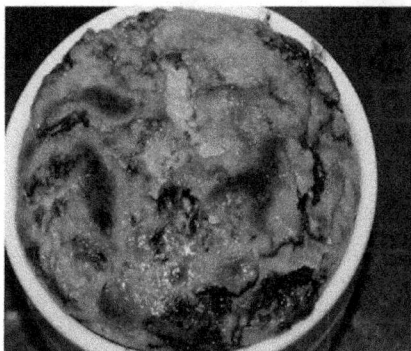

Coconut Flour Flaugnarde —pg 114

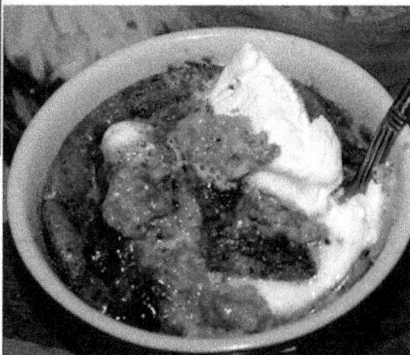

Cranberry Peach Cobbler—pg 116

Almond Tea Biscuits

A light and very tasty cookie made with a variety of flours. All cookies made with low carb flours tend to be delicate, so allow them plenty of time to cool before moving or storing. (Pictured on page 111.)

1/2 cup Almond Flour
1/2 cup Low Carb Flour
2 tablespoons Coconut Flour
1 tablespoon Vanilla Whey Protein Powder (optional)
1/4 teaspoon Baking Powder
1 teaspoon Cinnamon, ground
1/2 teaspoon Clove, ground
1 large Egg
1 teaspoon Almond Extract
3 tablespoons Almonds, sliced or flaked
1/2 cup Sugar Substitute

Preheat oven to 300 degrees.

In a medium bowl, mix together the flours, baking powder and cinnamon. Add egg, almond extract and sugar substitute. Stir together.

If the dough is too dry, add enough water to get a dough that will hold together. Let sit about five minutes for the coconut flour to absorb the liquid. If necessary, add a little more water and mix again to make a dough you can roll into balls.

Line a baking sheet with parchment paper. Take about a teaspoon of dough and roll into a ball. It should be about 3/4" in diameter. Place on cookie sheet and make the next one. You should get about 20 balls from the dough. Moisten your fingers and flatten the dough out into a 1 inch circle. If you wish, you can use a moistened fork to make little ridges in the cookie. Sprinkle almond flakes on each cookie or arrange almond slivers on each cookie to decorate.

Bake for 10 to 15 minutes until just barely turning brown.

Remove to cookie rack and let cool. Store in a plastic storage bag or other airtight container. Makes 20 cookies.

Nutrition Info per cookie
Calories: 38.4 Fat: 4.7 g Net Carbs: 0.9 g Protein: 1.6 g

Caramel Nut Cheesecake

I had a box or two of Atkin's Chocolate Caramel Nut bars that had gone past their expiration date by way more than a month and I wanted to do something with them. So I came up with this cheesecake recipe using the bars. You don't have to use a stale one; a fresh one works just fine. (Pictured on page 111.)

2 ounces Cream Cheese, softened
2 tablespoons Sugar Substitute
1 Atkins Chocolate Caramel Nut Bar
1 Egg
2 tablespoons Heavy Cream
1 tablespoons Coconut Flour or Whey Powder
1/2 teaspoon Vanilla

Preheat oven to 350 degrees (F). Prepare a muffin tin by spraying 4 wells with cooking spray or put in baking cups.

Chop the Carmel Nut bar into small pieces. In a small bowl, use a mixer to mix the cream cheese, vanilla, egg and sugar substitute together until creamy. Add in the whey powder or coconut flour and mix until all ingredients are blended. Hand stir in the Carmel Nut Bar pieces.

Spoon into the muffin cups, taking care to try to distribute the candy pieces evenly. Stirring the batter each time you dip out a spoonful will help.

Put a little water in the two empty muffin wells so you are not baking them empty. Bake for 20 to 25 minutes until a toothpick inserted in the middle of one comes out clean. Let cool before serving or refrigerate until about 30 minutes before you are ready to serve. To serve, put on a small plate or dessert bowl and top with a little sugar free chocolate syrup and a teaspoon of whipped cream, if you like.

Makes four mini-cheesecakes.

Nutrition Info per mini-cake:
Calories: 128.5 Fat: 11.5 g Net Carbs: 1.75 g Protein: 4.35 g

Coconut Flour Flaugnarde

I only discovered this yummy and easy to make dessert in the past couple of years and it quickly became a favorite. You can make it with almost any fresh fruit (I'd shy away from citrus fruits and melons), although the carb count will vary slightly with different fruits. This one uses blueberries or raspberries. Even though it is called a coconut flour version, you can also make it using almond flour or another low carb flour. If using one of the other flours, use 2 tablespoons of flour rather than the 1 of coconut flour. (Pictured on page 111.)

1/4 cup Blueberries or Raspberries
5 tablespoon Heavy Cream and 5 tablespoons Water
3 tablespoons Sugar Substitute
1 tablespoon Coconut Flour
2 Eggs
1 teaspoon Vanilla Extract or Almond Extract
1 teaspoon Butter, softened
Tiny pinch of Salt

Preheat oven to 425 degrees (F.) Butter two 1 cup ramekins.

Divide berries into ramekins, spreading evenly.

Blend milk, eggs, sugar, flour, and flavor extract until the batter is smooth. Pour over the berries and gently shake each ramekin to remove any air bubbles.

Bake until puffed and the center is set, about 25 minutes. Cool until the egg custard deflates, then serve warm with a tablespoon of whipped cream.

Nutrition Info per serving.
  Calories: 248 Fat: 20.9 g Net Carbs: 4.8 g Protein: 7.7 g

Cranberry Pumpkin Biscotti Cookies

Biscotti cookies aren't as hard to make as you might think, but they do take a little time to prepare. I've used a combination of flours and Vanilla whey protein powder to make mine, but you can just use 1 cup of low carb flour total to replace both the coconut flour and the whey powder. Don't use all coconut flour or all almond flour as they won't hold together as well. (Pictured on page 111.)

1 tablespoons Extra Virgin Olive Oil
2 tablespoons Sugar Substitute
1 tablespoons Brown Sugar Substitute
1/2 teaspoon Vanilla Extract
1/2 tablespoon Pumpkin Spice Syrup
1 large Egg
3 tablespoons Pumpkin puree
1 1/4 teaspoons ground Cinnamon
1/2 teaspoon ground Clove (optional)
3 tablespoons Low Carb Flour
2 tablespoons Coconut Flour
1 1/2 tablespoons Vanilla Whey Protein Powder
1/2 teaspoon Baking Powder
1/2 teaspoon Baking Soda
1/4 cup Cranberries, chopped
1/4 cup Pecans or Walnuts, chopped

Preheat the oven to 300 degrees (F).

In a large bowl, mix together oil and sugar until well blended. Mix in the vanilla and almond extracts, then beat in the eggs. Combine flour, salt, and baking powder; gradually stir into egg mixture. Mix in cranberries and nuts by hand.

Divide dough in half. Form two logs (12x2 inches) on a cookie sheet that has been lined with parchment paper. Dough may be sticky; wet hands with cool water to handle dough more easily.

Bake for 35 minutes in the preheated oven, or until logs are light brown. Remove from oven, and set aside to cool for 10 minutes. Reduce oven heat to 275 degrees (F).

Cut logs on a diagonal into 3/4 inch thick slices. Lay on sides on parchment covered cookie sheet. Bake approximately 8 to 10 minutes, or until dry; cool.

Makes 12 cookies

Nutrition per cookie
  Calories: 46.9 Total Fat: 3.9 g Net Carbs: 1.0 g Protein: 1.3 g

Cranberry Peach Cobbler

This a quick recipe to make and brings together the great taste of peaches and cranberries. Cobblers are simply fresh fruit sprinkled with sugar and seasonings with a biscuit crust on top. So satisfying though. Add a little fresh cream or whipped cream on top. (Pictured on page 111.)

1/4 cup fresh Peach slices
1/4 cup fresh Cranberries, chopped
1/2 tablespoon Butter
2 tablespoon Pecans, chopped (optional)
3 tablespoons Low Carb Flour or Almond Flour
1/4 teaspoon Baking Powder
1 tablespoon Heavy Cream
1 tablespoon Water
1/2 teaspoon Cinnamon
1/4 cup Sugar Substitute, divided
1 teaspoon granulated Sugar Substitute for the crust

Makes 2

Preheat oven to 365 degrees F.

Split butter between two 1/2 cup ramekins. Put in microwave for about 20 seconds to melt the butter or put in hot oven for about 5 minutes.

Add the peaches, cranberries, sugar substitute, pecans and seasonings to a small bowl and mix together. Microwave for 1 minute to heat up. Or you can put the fruit, sugar substitute and nuts into a pan and heat on the stove, stirring a little, until hot. Spoon 1/2 of the mixture in each of the ramekins.

Mix the flour and baking powder together. Add cream, water, a teaspoon of sugar substitute and stir well. If dough is too thick to spread, add a little more water. Spread dough on top of the fruit in the ramekin.

Bake for 15 to 18 minutes until the crust is browned. Let cool a few minutes, then serve with whipped cream or just a little cream poured over the top.

Makes two cobblers.

Nutrition Info per cobbler:
Calories:168 Fat:13.5 g Net Carbs: 6.6 g Protein: 5.2 g

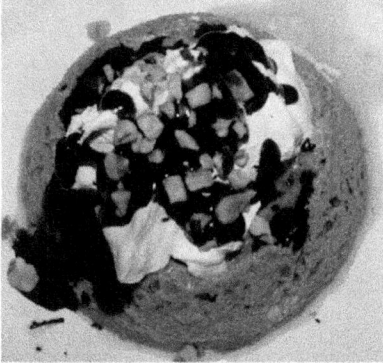

Espresso Hazelnut Custard
with Bourbon Sauce—pg 119

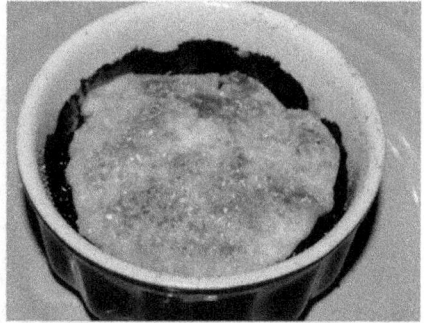

Blueberry Dumpling—pg 120

Peanut Butter
Blossom Cookies—pg 121

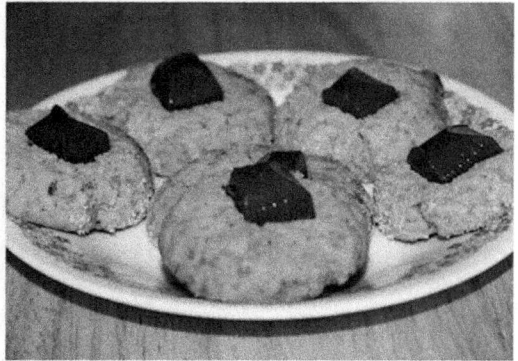

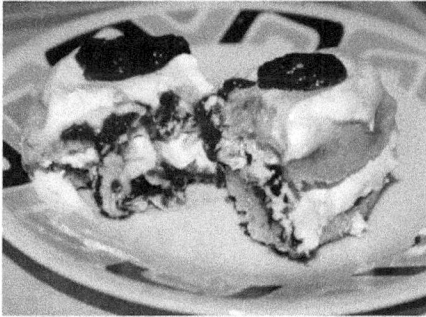

Raspberry Lemon Drop Torte—pg 123

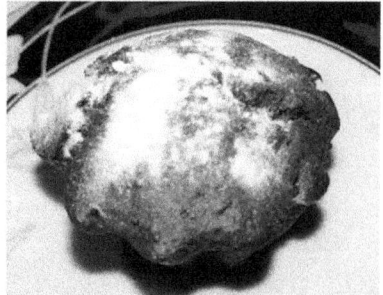

Peanut Butter Chocolate Cake—pg 122

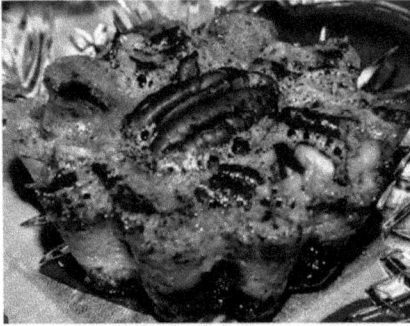

Cranberry Chocolate Pecan Tartlets—pg 125

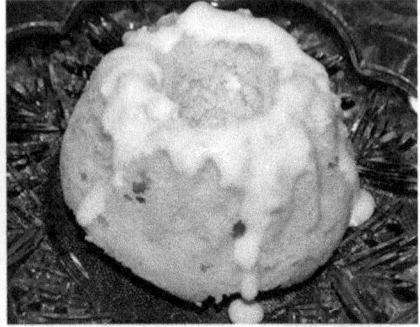

Sour Cream Lemon Cake—pg 124

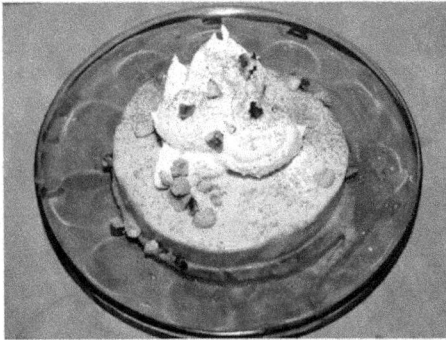

Pumpkin Flan—pg 127

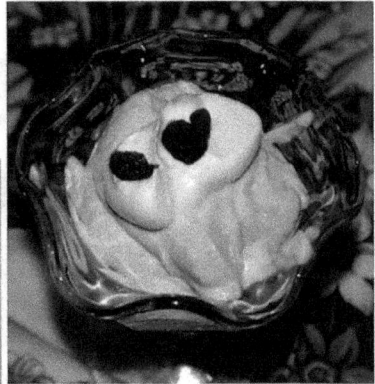

Pumpkin Cheese Mousse—pg 126

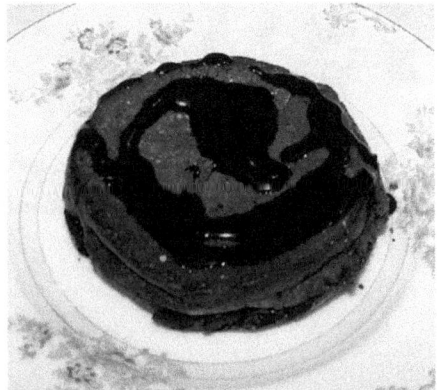

Chocolate Mist Cheesecake—pg 128

Espresso Hazelnut Custard & Bourbon Sauce

An elegant, yet light dessert for two. Very satisfying after a heavy meal. (Pictured on page 117.)

Custard
1/2 cup Heavy Cream
¼ cup Cold Water
1 teaspoon Espresso Instant Powdered Coffee
2 tablespoons Sugar Substitute
1 teaspoon Sugar Free Hazelnut Syrup
1 Egg

Sauce
1 oz Bourbon
2 tablespoon Brown Sugar Substitute
1 teaspoon Butter

Garnish
1 tablespoon whipped cream
1 tablespoon ground hazelnuts

Prepare two 6 oz cups or ramekins by buttering the bottom and sides lightly or spray with a cooking spray.

In a small bowl, beat the egg with a wire whip, then add the cream, sugar, coffee and hazelnut syrup. Beat until the coffee is completely dissolved. Split the egg mixture equally between the two cups.

In a deep skillet, add water, put the cups into the water and add additional water to the skillet to bring the water line outside the cups up to 1/2" from the top of the cups. Bring the water to a boil, then turn it to low and put a lid or foil over the top of the skillet. Simmer for 10 to 15 minutes until the custard is set.

Remove from the pan using tongs or a padded glove to prevent burning your hand. Cover each custard with plastic wrap, allowing it to sit on top of the custard. This will help prevent a film from forming. Put in the refrigerator for at least three hours.

When ready to serve, put the butter, bourbon and brown sugar substitute into a small sauce pan and cook until it begins to thicken.

Unmold the custard, if you wish, or serve in the cup with a tablespoon of sauce over the top, and a spoon of whipped cream. Garnish with ground hazelnuts.

Nutrition Info per serving:
Calories: 310.6 Fat: 6.1g Net Carbs: 2.5 g Protein: 4.7 g

Blueberry Dumplings

Quick and easy to make, these dumplings use a little low carb flour and a few blueberries to make a special dessert that tastes fabulous. (Pictured on page 117.)

1/4 cup Blueberries
1/4 cup Low Carb Flour or Almond Flour
1 teaspoon Water
1 tablespoon Shortening or Butter
1/2 teaspoon Almond Extract
1 tablespoon Almonds, chopped (Optional)
2 tablespoons Granulated Sugar Substitute

Preheat oven to 425 degrees (F.)

Mix the pastry dough by combining 1/4 cup low carb flour with 1 tablespoon shortening or butter and mix with a fork (or your fingers) to make a crumbly dough. Add 1 teaspoon of water and continue mixing, pulling the dough together until it forms a pie dough. Put a little almond flour or coconut flour on a board. Cut the dough in two and pat one section into a round. Use a small roller to roll into a flat circle large enough to fit the top of the ramekin. Repeat with the second dough section.

Spray two 1/2 cup ramekins with cooking spray. Put half the blueberries into each ramekin. Sprinkle almond extract and sugar substitute on top of the blueberries, half to each ramekin. Add almonds, if you wish. Fit the pie dough on top of the peaches. Allow space for the juices to bubble up. Sprinkle a little sugar substitute on top of each dumpling.

Bake for 20 to 25 minutes until crust is golden brown. Makes 2 servings.

Nutrition Info per serving (with almonds)
Calories: 129 Fat: 10.8 g Net Carbs: 4.3 g Protein: 3.8 g

Peanut Butter Blossom Cookies

You can have delicious peanut butter cookies when you make them with low carb flours. This uses three flours to make sturdy cookies. If you don't like coconut flour, then substitute in 2 tablespoons more of almond flour. (Pictured on page 117.)

12 Sugar free Candy Kisses
    or 6 Russell Stover's Chocolate Miniatures*
1/4 cup Butter Flavored Shortening
1/3 cup JIF Creamy Peanut Butter
3 tablespoons Sugar Substitute
3 tablespoons Brown Sugar Substitute
1 Egg
1 tablespoon Heavy Cream
1/2 teaspoon Vanilla Extract
2 tablespoons Low Carb Flour
2 tablespoons Almond Flour
1 tablespoon Coconut Flour
2 tablespoons Vanilla Whey Protein Powder
1 teaspoon Baking Soda
1/4 teaspoon Salt
1/2 teaspoon Cinnamon
Additional granulated Sugar Substitute

Heat oven to 375 degrees F. Remove wrappers from chocolates. If using chocolate miniatures, cut each in half with a sharp knife warmed in hot water.

Beat shortening and peanut butter in a bowl until well blended. Add both sugar substitutes, beat until fluffy. Add egg, cream, water and vanilla; beat well. Stir dry ingredients together and gradually beat into peanut butter mixture.

Shape dough into 12 one inch balls, about the size of a walnut in the shell. Roll in sugar and place on ungreased cookie sheet.

Bake 8 to 10 minutes or until lightly browned. Immediately press a chocolate into the center of each cookie. Cookie will crack around the edges. Remove from cookie sheet to wire rack. Cool completely.

Nutrition per cookie based on 1 dozen.
   Calories: 96 Fat: 9.0 g Net Carbs: 1.8 g Protein: 2.4 g

*I used Russell Stover's sugar free miniatures solid chocolate candy cut in half. It is the lowest carb that I've found for chocolates with 0 net carbs in a serving of 5. Calories for 5 are 190. You only use 1/2 chocolate piece per cookie.

Peanut Butter Chocolate Cake

Of all the nut flours I've used, only peanut flour has a strong taste of the nut from which it was created. So, it's ideal for making peanut butter-type baked goodies, like peanut butter cookies and this peanut butter chocolate cake. (Pictured on page 117.)

3 tablespoons Low Carb Flour
2 tablespoons Peanut Flour
2 tablespoons Crunchy Peanut Butter
2 tablespoons Butter, soft
2 tablespoons Unsweetened Cocoa Powder
1/2 teaspoon Baking Powder
1 Egg
2 tablespoons Coconut Milk or Heavy Cream
1 tablespoon Water
1/2 cup Sugar Substitute
1/4 cup Sugar Free Chocolate Chips

Preheat oven to 350 degrees F.

Prepare a small 3" cake pan or aluminum individual pot pie tin by spraying with cooking spray.

In a bowl, mix flours, baking powder and butter together. Add egg, cream and water and stir well to make a smooth batter. Pour into the pan or tin and smooth to make an even top. Sprinkle chocolate chips over the top.

Bake for about 15 minutes. Test with a toothpick, which should come out clean when poked in the middle of the cake. If it is still gooey, cook a few minutes longer and retest.

Let cool, then flip cake out of the pan and turn over on a plate. Dust top with about 1/2 teaspoon of confectioner's sugar substitute. (You can make your own by processing sugar substitute in a food processor until it is a powder.)

Makes 4 cupcakes.

Nutrition Info per cupcake
Calories: 180 Fat: 15.8 g Net Carbs: 4.3 g Protein: 6.7 g

Raspberry Lemon Drop Tart

This elegant, wonderful blend of flavor dessert was inspired by one at a chain restaurant that was too high carb'd to even consider. But it does convert to a low carb version pretty easily. Preparation can be done a few hours before serving time with the assembly taking place no more than two hours before to keep it fresh. (Pictured on page 117.)

1 Sour Cream Lemon Cake (recipe follows on next page)
2 tablespoons Sugar Free Raspberry Jam

Lemon curd
3 Eggs
1/2 cup plus 2 tablespoons Sugar Substitute
1/3 cup Lemon Juice
1/4 cup Butter
2 teaspoons Lemon Pulp

Whipped cream or use Cool Whip
1/8 cup Heavy Whipping Cream, chilled
1 oz. Cream Cheese
1 teaspoon Sugar Substitute
1/4 teaspoon Vanilla

Make the lemon curd. Bring water to a boil in the lower pan of a double boiler or in the larger of two pots that will stack one in the other. Reduce to a simmer and whisk eggs, sugar and lemon juice in the top pot until it's mixed well. Break any lumps in the mixture as you are stirring. Continue stirring until it thickens, about 8 to 10 minutes. If there are lumps, press through a mesh strainer to remove them. Fold in butter until it is completely mixed into the curd. Mix in the lemon zest and chill in the refrigerator for 4 hours. You will have extra lemon curd. Put in a jar, refrigerate and use with scones, muffins or toast.

Starting with cold whipping cream, whip to peaks. In a separate bowl, mix the cream cheese with 1 tablespoon sugar substitute and 1 teaspoon vanilla in a blender or with egg beaters. Save 1 tablespoons of the whipped cream for decoration and mix the rest with the cream cheese mixture, folding it in until it is completely mixed.

Assemble the cake shortly before serving: you can make it before dinner and refrigerate a couple of hours, but don't let sit too long. Cut the mini yellow cake in half across the height using a sharp knife.

Spread half the whipped cream cheese on the bottom. Spoon half the raspberry jam on top of cream cheese. Top with the other half of the yellow cake and spread another layer of whipped cream cheese. Spread 2 tablespoons of lemon curd on top of cream cheese. Put a dollop of raspberry jam in the center and make drops of whipped cream around it by dropping it off a small spoon.

Refrigerate until ready to serve. Cut into quarters and serve two quarters per serving. Makes 2 servings.

Nutrition Info per tablespoon Lemon Curd – makes about 16 tablespoons
  Calories: 42.8   Fat: 3.8 g   Net Carbs: 0.8 g   Protein: 1.3 g

Nutrition Info per serving with cake:
  Calories: 284.7   Fat: 25.3 g   Net Carbs: 7.1 g   Protein: 6.4 g

Sour Cream Lemon Cake

Thanks to a little sugar free lemon pudding in the mix, this cake is very moist and filled with lemon flavor. (Pictured on page 118.)

1/2 cup Low Carb Flour
2 tablespoons Coconut Flour
1 tablespoon Lemon Sugar Free Pudding Mix
1 teaspoon Baking Powder
Dash Salt
2 tablespoons Sour Cream
1 tablespoon Lemon Juice
1/4 cup Sugar Substitute
1 large Egg
2 tablespoons Egg White
1/4 cup Butter, melted

Icing
1/4 cup Confectioners' Sugar Substitute
1 tablespoon Sour Cream
1 tablespoon Heavy Cream

Preheat oven to 350 degrees (F.) Prepare three 3-inch cake molds or 3 cleaned tuna fish cans by lining bottoms with parchment paper and spraying the sides. Or spray 6 cupcake molds to make individual cakes.

In a small bowl, mix all the dry ingredients, except sugar substitute, together. In a larger bowl, use a mixer to combine the rest of the ingredients together, adding the lemon juice last. Add the dry ingredients about 1/3 at a time and mix well.

Spoon or pour the batter into the prepared cupcake molds. Bake for 20 to 25 minutes until the center springs back when pressed. Let cool for about 10 minutes before removing from mold, then let cool completely before icing.

To make icing, use a mixer to combine icing ingredients until smooth. Add enough water, if needed, to make a sauce consistency, then drizzle on the cakes. Makes 6 servings.

Nutrition Info per serving:
  Calories: 137   Fat:17.8 g   Net Carbs: 3.7 g   Protein: 3.7 g

Note: Use one 3" cake to make the Raspberry Lemon Drop Torte. I used Smuckers Sugar Free Raspberry Preserves for it.

Cranberry Chocolate Pecan Pie Tarts

This is my own variation on the southern Pecan Pie. I love cranberries and chocolate, so it seemed like a great innovation to add them to a pecan pie. The small tarts are a great serving control with this rich-tasting pie and they look very elegant for dessert. (Pictured on page 118.)

1 Egg
1/4 cup Sugar Free Maple Syrup
1/4 cup Sugar Substitute
1/4 cup Pecans, broken into pieces
4 Pecan halves for topping
1/2 teaspoon Vanilla
1/2 teaspoon Cinnamon, ground
2 tablespoons Sugar Free Chocolate Chips
1/4 cup Sugar Free Cranberry Jam (see Note)
Pinch salt

Crumble Dough
2 tablespoons Almond Flour
1 1/2 teaspoons Butter, softened
1/2 tablespoon Sugar Substitute

Preheat oven to 350 degrees (f.) Prepare four silicon tart cups (muffin sized) by spraying with baking spray. Tarts with straight edges are easier to unmold. Or you can put paper cups in regular-sized muffin wells.

Mix the crust first. Combine ingredients in a small bowl and mix with a fork until it is pulling together but still in crumbles. Press about 1 tablespoon into the bottom of each of the tart cups. Bake for about 10 minutes to set the crust and lightly brown it.

While crust is baking, make the filling. Combine the eggs, maple syrup, sugar substitute, vanilla, salt and cinnamon in a bowl and mix together, then add slightly cooled melted butter. Stir in the broken pecans and mix well.

Remove pans from the oven, then distribute the chocolate chips evenly in each of the cups, about 1/2 tablespoon per cup. Add 1 tablespoon Cranberry Jam on top of the chocolate chips and spread to cover the top. Divide the pecan filling into the eight cups, about 2 to 2 1/2 tablespoons per cup. Top with a pecan half on each tart.

Bake for 35 minutes. Let cool for about 15 minutes before servings. Add a little whipped cream or Cool Whip if you like. Makes 4 servings

Nutrition Info per tart
  Calories: 166.3 Fat: 14.5g Net Carbs: 2.2g Protein: 3.7g

Note: To make sugar free Cranberry Jam, follow the instructions on the Cranberry package to make Cranberry sauce, using sugar substitute for the sugar, add 1 teaspoon of pectin and cook for about 20 minutes after the cranberries pop. Let cool and store in a jar for about a month. You can also freeze it into smaller portions and thaw as needed.

Rene Averett

Pumpkin Cheese Mousse

An easy dessert to make and it so refreshing. Have a nice cup of coffee or tea with this and it'll end your meal perfectly. The low carb version uses Carbmasters Cultured Dairy Blend from Kroger Foods, which is like yogurt and is 4 net carbs for the whole 6 oz. If it isn't available, look for the lowest carb Greek yogurt you can find to keep the carbs and calories down. (Pictured on page 118.)

3 ounces Yogurt or Dairy Blend
2 tablespoons Pumpkin puree
2 tablespoons Cream Cheese
1/2 teaspoon Pumpkin Pie spice
2 tablespoons whipped topping
2 teaspoons Reduced Sugar Crasins, chopped
2 Reduced Sugar Crasins for topping
2 sprigs fresh Mint

In a small bowl, add the dairy blend or yogurt, pumpkin, creamed cheese and pumpkin pie spice and mix together well with a hand mixer or beat with a spoon to get the cream cheese and pumpkin blended in well. Save 2 teaspoons of whipped topping then add the rest and the chopped crasins to the yogurt and mix until blended.

Spoon evenly into two serving glasses or small bowls, cover with plastic wrap and refrigerate until ready to serve. Just before serving, put 1 teaspoon of whipped topping on each and garnish with the reserved crasins and a sprig of mint.

Makes 2 servings.

Nutrition Info per serving using 3 net carbs per 3 oz. serving yogurt:
Calories: 100.8   Fat: 5.7 g   Net Carbs: 6.8 g   Protein: 5.0 g

Pumpkin Flan

Basically a baked caramel egg custard, flan is a light, low carb and very tasty dessert. It is also easy to make. This version uses sugar free maple syrup as a substitute for brown sugar syrup and adds pumpkin to it. Ideally, the custard will not have any bubbles on the sides when it is cooked, but with almond milk or coconut milk, it is harder to achieve the smooth finish. (Pictured on page 118.)

1/4 cup Sugar Free Maple Syrup
1 large Egg
2 tablespoons Sugar Substitute
1/4 cup Pumpkin Puree
1 1/4 teaspoon Pumpkin Pie Spice
1/2 teaspoon Vanilla
Pinch salt
1/2 cup Almond Milk or Coconut Milk or heavy cream

Preheat oven to 300 degrees.

Butter or spray two one 1/2 cup ramekins, put 1 tablespoon of the syrup in each and roll around the bottoms to coat ramekins. Mix the remaining ingredients together until smooth. Pour into ramekins, dividing mixture evenly to about 1/2 inch from the top. Put ramekins into a shallow pan with about 1 inch of water in it. Bake for 45 to 50 minutes or until the custard is set. Chill for at least 4 hours before serving. Garnish with a dollop of whipped cream or cool whip.

Nutrition Info with almond or coconut milk:
Calories: 59 Fat: 3.2 g Net Carbs: 2.4 g Protein: 3.8

Nutrition Info with heavy cream:
Calories: 256.8 Fat: 24.6 g Net Carbs: 4.1 g Protein: 4.8 g

Chocolate Mist Cheesecake

The perfect treat when you want a bit of chocolate to end your evening. This recipe is easy and cooks quickly, just 15 to 20 minutes in the oven or toaster oven (add 5 more minutes for the toaster oven). The Irish Mist in it brings a light whiskey flavor to the dessert. Fair warning though, it does add a few carbs to the cake. You can make this without the Irish Mist and it will be about 2.5 fewer carbs. Makes 2 personal cheesecakes. To be honest, I usually cut one in half because it's that rich! (Pictured on page 118.)

2 oz Cream Cheese
3 tablespoon Sugar Substitute
1 Egg
2 tablespoons Heavy Cream
1 tablespoon Cocoa Powder
1/2 teaspoon Vanilla
1 tablespoon Irish Mist (optional)

Preheat oven to 350 degrees (F).

Butter, or spray with cooking spray, two 1 cup ramekins or two small oven safe dessert bowls.

In a small bowl, use a mixer to blend the cream cheese, vanilla and sugar substitute together. Stir in the egg, cream, Irish mist and cocoa powder until all ingredients are moistened, then mix well with beaters.

Put 1/2 of the batter into each ramekin. Place ramekins on a baking sheet and bake for 15 to 20 minutes until a toothpick inserted in the middle comes out clean. Let cool for about 20 minutes before serving. Pour a little sugar free chocolate syrup over the top, add a strawberry and add a dollop of whipped cream or cool whip, if you'd like.

Makes 2 large servings or 4 smaller servings.

Nutrition Info per serving (with Irish mist and chocolate chips):
Calories: 222 Fat: 17.8 g Net Carbs: 7.7 g Protein: 5.7 g

Hint: If you wish, you can make four servings in cupcake molds. If you use silicone molds, they will come out of the mold easier.

Breads

T'is said that man does not live by bread alone, but neither does he live happily without it. It's true that regular bread, delicious though it is, has way more starches and carbs than we want in our meals. Luckily, there are some low carb flour options on the market and even some baking mixes. Using these, some of which are available at most grocery stores, you can make a variety of breads to satisfy that longing.

Baked Low Carb Crumpets   130
Baked Tortilla Chips   131
Cream Cheese Biscuit   132
Peanut Butter Surprise Muffin   133
Flat Bread Crackers   134
Flax Meal Muffin or Roll   137
Irish Soda Bread   138
Greek Yogurt Muffin   139
Simple Crepes   140
Cheese Taco Shells   141
Flax Meal Focaccia Bread   142

Baked Low Carb Crumpets

A variation on a basic muffin recipe. By adding yeast and adjusting the flours slightly, you get a very nice version of a crumpet that is satisfying and toasty as well as low in carbs and calories. This works great as the base for Eggs Benedict. (Pictured on page 135.)

1/4 cup Low Carb Flour
1/4 cup Almond Flour
1 tablespoon Coconut Flour
1 package Active Dry Yeast
2 tablespoons Buttermilk
1 large Egg
1/2 tablespoon Shortening
1/8 teaspoon Salt
2 tablespoons warm Water
1 teaspoon Sugar Substitute

You will need four 3" round molds to make these. You can use cleaned and greased tuna or other 3" short cans. Grease the sides of the rings.

Preheat oven to 365 degrees (F.)

Put warm water in a small cup and sprinkle yeast over the top. Add sugar substitute and stir in. Let sit for about five minutes to activate the yeast.

In a bowl, mix the flours and salt with the shortening, cutting through with two knives or a pastry cutter until the mixture is crumbly. Add the egg, buttermilk and yeast and mix together with a spoon. It should make a thick batter rather than a dough. If it is too dry, add a little warm water. Let sit in a warm spot for at least 30 minutes. Stir down the batter.

Place the molds on a baking sheet. Spoon the batter into the rings. Bake for 15 to 18 minutes until the crumpets are golden brown.

Nutrition Info per crumpet
Calories: 113 Fat: 7.9 g Net Carbs: 3.0 g Protein: 5.0 g

Baked Tortilla Chips

Not a recipe to make flour tortillas – perhaps in another cookbook – but to use commercial low carb tortillas to make chips for dipping. (Pictured on page 135.)

Makes 32 chips

2 low carb Tortillas, 6" (3 nc each)
1 tablespoon Butter, melted

Preheat oven or toaster oven to 375 degrees (F.) Prepare a cookie sheet with parchment paper sprayed with cooking spray.

Cut tortillas into 8 triangular wedges. Cut tortilla in half, then cut or cut into quarters. Cut each quarter into four triangles as shown below. Arrange tortilla triangles on baking sheet and brush with melted butter or spray with butter flavored cooking spray.

Bake for 10 minutes or until the tortillas are toasted. Let cool, then store in an airtight can or use.

Nutrition Info per serving (8 chips to a serving) La Tortilla Factory

Nutrition Info per serving (8 chips to a serving) Mama Lupe's
   Calories: 30 Fat: 1.5 g Net Carbs: 1.5 g Protein: 2.5 g

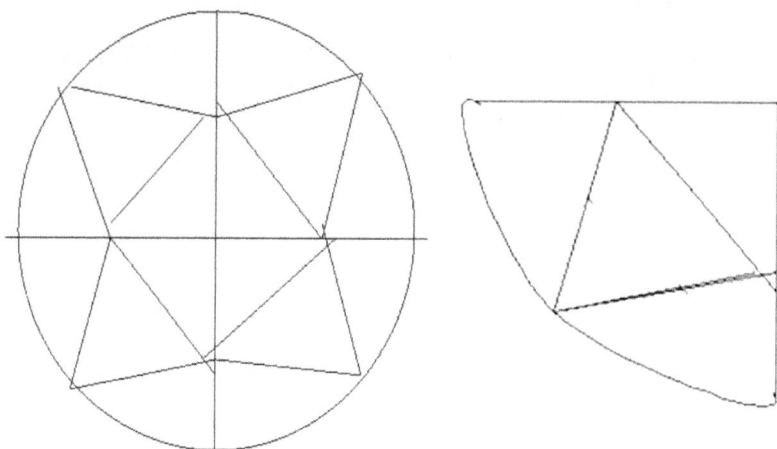

Cream Cheese Biscuit

Delicious, tasty muffin-like biscuits. Use them for sandwiches or as a biscuit. (Pictured on page 135.)

3/4 cup Low Carb Flour
1 tablespoon Oat Fiber (optional)
Pinch Salt
1/2 tablespoon Baking Powder
1/2 teaspoon Garlic powder
1 teaspoon Sugar Substitute
2 tablespoons Olive Oil
2 large Eggs
1/2 tablespoon Dried Onion Flakes
3 ounces Cream Cheese

Heat oven to 360 degrees F.

In a bowl, mix low carb flour, oat fiber, salt, garlic powder and baking powder together.

In a larger bowl, use a mixer to mix the cream cheese, then add eggs, oil and sucralose or sugar substitute. Add dry ingredients gradually. When mixture gets thick, clean off the egg beaters and stir in the onion flakes with a spoon and enough water to make a sticky dough.

Spray a baking pan or round molds with cooking spray and divide equally into the molds or drop about two tablespoons on the baking pan and shape into rounds.

Bake for about 20 minutes until golden brown. Makes 3 large biscuits or 4 smaller ones.

Nutrition Info per biscuit
Calories: 352.5 Fat: 32 Net Carbs: 4.6 g Protein: 5.3 g

Peanut Butter Surprise Muffin

A simple to make and fun muffin with the peanut butter and jam on the inside. Makes a nice Sunday brunch treat. You can use Half and Half instead of the heavy cream or even substitute Almond Milk for the cream and water.

2 tablespoons Peanut Flour or Almond Flour
1 tablespoons Coconut flour or 2 tablespoons low carb flour
1 Egg
1 Egg White
1/2 teaspoon Baking Powder
1/2 teaspoon Cinnamon, ground
2 tablespoons Coconut Oil
1/2 teaspoon Vanilla Extract
1 teaspoon Heavy Whipping Cream
1 teaspoon Water
1 tablespoons JIF creamy peanut butter
2 teaspoons Low Carb Strawberry Jam

Preheat oven to 360 degrees F. Prepare two muffin cups with baking spray. Solo muffin cups are best for this. If you use a pan that has six wells, put water in the other wells before baking.

Mix flours and baking powder together and add the cinnamon. Beat eggs, whipping cream, water and vanilla extract together with a fork, then stir in coconut oil and mix into flours. Combine until moist, but don't over mix. If the mixture is too dry, add a little water until it is a droppable consistency.

Using 1/2 of the batter, fill each muffin cup about 1/3 full. Spoon half the peanut butter into the middle of each muffin on top of the batter and top with a teaspoon of strawberry jam. Divide the remainder of the batter equally over the top of the filling mixture.

Bake for about 20 minutes until the muffin is golden brown. Cool and serve. Makes 2 muffins.

Nutrition Info per muffin
Calories 187.8, Net Carbs: 5.1 g, Protein: 10.3 g

Flat Bread Crackers

This is a simple cracker that you can use with spreads, cold cuts, or other typical cracker items. I use wheat germ in mine for extra flavor and nutrition, but you can omit it. Add an extra tablespoon of flax meal if you leave it out. You can use regular flax meal or golden flax or a combination. (Pictured on page 135.)

1/4 cup Almond Flour
1/4 cup Flax Meal
1 teaspoon Garlic Powder
1/2 teaspoon Baking Powder
1/4 teaspoon Salt
1 tablespoon Wheat Germ (optional)
1 tablespoon Coconut Oil or Olive Oil
1/2 teaspoon Sugar Substitute

Preheat oven to 365 degrees (F.) Coat a cookie sheet with cooking spray or cover the pan with parchment paper and spray the paper.

Mix all ingredients together and add enough water to make a thick paste-like dough. Put half the dough onto one end of the pan and shape it into a 4"x4" square. Smooth the edges as much as possible and try to make the top even. Repeat with the other half of the dough.

Bake for 15 minutes until the flat bread is cooked and lightly browned. Let cool for 5 minutes, then cut each square into quarters.

Makes 8 crackers or 2 servings.

Nutrition Information per cracker
Calories: 21.6 Fat: 1.8 g Net Carbs: 0.3 g Protein: 0.9 g

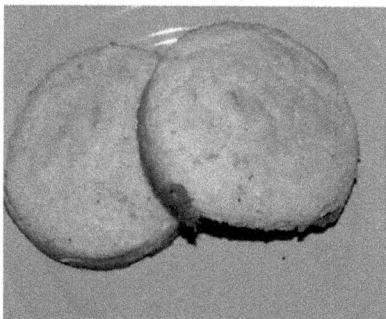

Baked Crumpets—pg 130

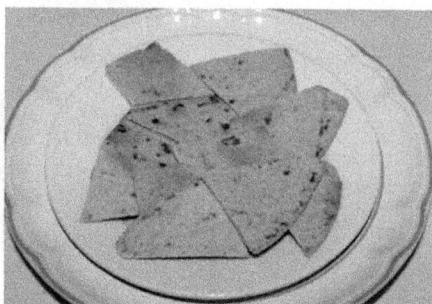

Baked Tortilla Chips—pg 131

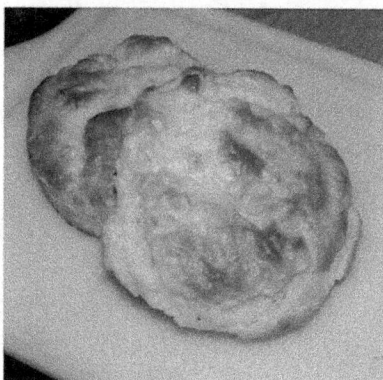

Cream Cheese Biscuit—pg 132

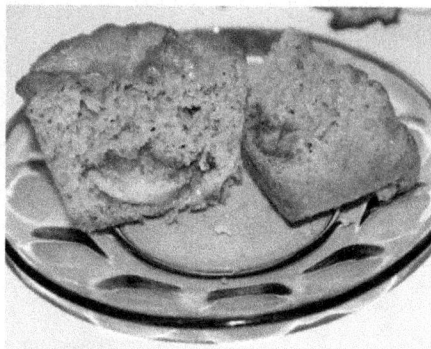

Peanut Butter & Jam Surprise Muffin—pg 133

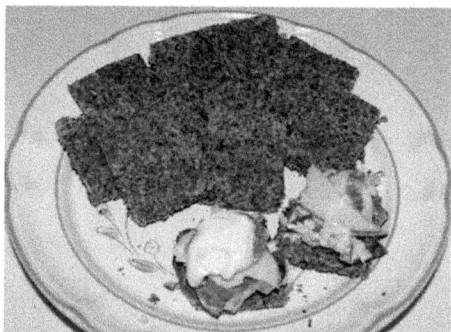

Flat Bread Crackers— pg 134

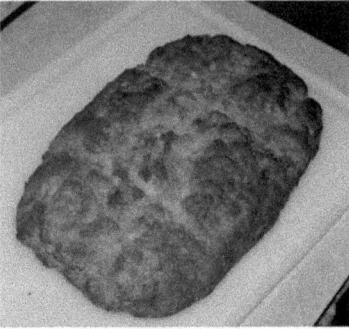

Irish Soda Bread—pg 138

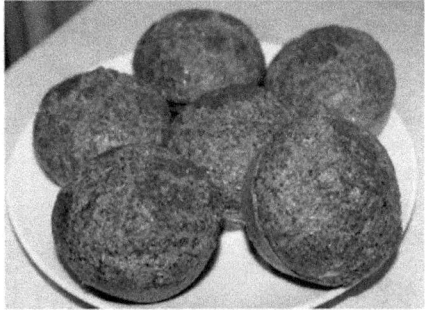

Flax Meal Rolls—pg 137

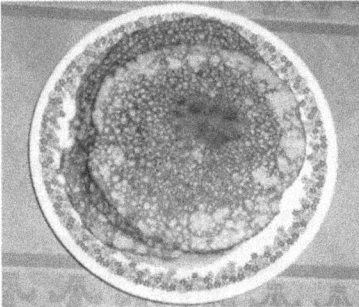

Simple Crepes—pg 140

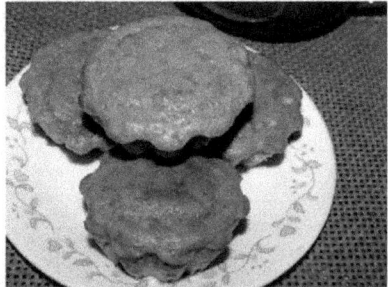

Greek Yogurt Muffins—pg 139

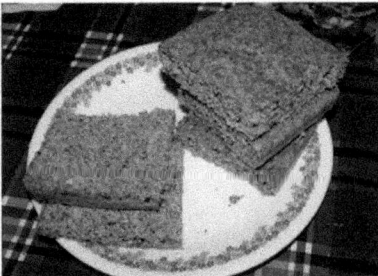

Flax Meal Focaccia Bread-page142

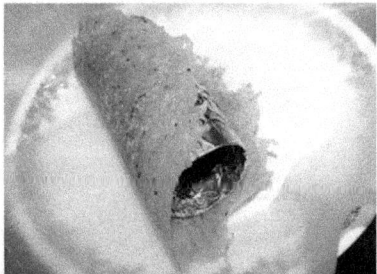

Cheese Taco Shells—pg 141

Flax Meal Muffin or Roll

This is a slight variation on Atkins' Muffin in a Minute recipe. It makes a tasty baked muffin or roll rather than a microwave one. Flax meal is terrific on a low carb plan since the fiber in it cancels out any carbohydrates. This makes for a great low carb bread. The taste is a bit nutty. You either like it or you don't. I'm offering the sweet version with cinnamon and you can add additional sweetener if you'd like. It works well with butter and low carb jams. The savory version uses Parmesan cheese and you can add garlic powder if you'd like a little more flavor. Good with soups and salads. (Pictured on page 136.)

1/4 cup Ground Flax Meal
1/2 teaspoons Baking Powder
Pinch Salt
1teaspoon Sugar substitute
1 large Egg
1 tablespoon Olive Oil
1 teaspoon ground Cinnamon or
2 teaspoons grated Parmesan Cheese

Preheat oven to 355 degrees (F.) Spray two 1/2 cup ramekins with baking spray.

In a bowl, mix together the wet ingredients, then add the rest of the ingredients and mix well. Make sure the egg is completely mixed in.

Divide the batter into the two ramekins. Bake for 15 to 18 minutes until a toothpick inserted in the middle comes out clean. Remove and cool a few minutes before eating.

Makes 2.

Nutrition Info per muffin
  Calories: 130 Fat: 9.2 g Net carbs: 0.8 g Protein: 6.2 g

Rene Averett

Irish Soda Bread

One of the first breads I made when I started converting recipes to low carb. This is easy and tastes great. It's similar to a biscuit dough and is very flavorful. Wonderful with soups and stews. (Pictured on page 136.)

1 1/4 cups Low Carb Flour
1 teaspoons Baking Powder
1 teaspoon Baking Soda
2 teaspoons Sugar substitute
2 tablespoons Butter, softened
1 large Egg
1/3 cup Buttermilk

Preheat oven to 375 degrees F (190 degrees C). Lightly grease a baking sheet.

In a large bowl, cut together or use your clean fingers to mix flour, sugar, baking soda, baking powder, salt and butter until you get pea-sized crumbles. Mix in buttermilk and egg. Turn dough out onto a lightly floured, using low carb flour, surface and knead slightly. Form dough into a round and place on prepared baking sheet. Use a sharp knife to cut an 'X' into the top of the loaf.

Bake in preheated oven for 40 to 50 minutes, or until a toothpick inserted into the center of the loaf comes out clean, You may continue to brush the loaf with the butter while it bakes.

Makes 6 slices or wedges

Nutrition Info per slice
Calories: 108 Fat: 8.5 g Net Carbs: 2.2 g Protein: 5.3 g

Greek Yogurt Muffin

This makes a nice, spiced breakfast muffin that goes great with just butter or even a little sugar free jam on it.

The Greek yogurt adds a new flavor and texture to it. Look for the lowest carb yogurt you can find. It helps to give the muffins a lift and adds texture. Peanut flour will add a slight peanut taste or you can use almond flour instead. The coconut flour will absorb more liquid, so if you substitute it with almond flour, use 4 tablespoons to replace the 2 of coconut flour. The clove is optional. While I love the taste of it, not everyone is so enchanted. (Pictured on page 136.)

1/4 cup Low Carb Flour
2 tablespoons Coconut Flour
1/4 cup light Peanut Flour or Almond Flour
1 large Egg
1/4 cup Greek Yogurt
1 teaspoon Baking Powder
1 Egg White (liquid is fine)
1 teaspoon Oil
1 tablespoon ground Cinnamon
1 teaspoon ground Clove (optional)
1 teaspoon Vanilla Extract

Preheat oven to 365 degrees (F.) Prepare a 6 well muffin pan by spraying with baking spray.

In a small bowl, mix the flours and baking powder together. In a larger bowl, mix together the yogurt, egg, egg white and vanilla until blended smoothly. Add the seasonings and oil, then add the flour, mixing until combined.

Spoon into muffin wells, distributing the batter equally. Bake for 18 to 20 minutes until golden brown and the center springs back when pressed. Let cool a few minutes before eating.

Makes 6 muffins.

Nutrition Info per muffin
  Calories: 98 Fat : 6.1 g Net Carbs: 3.3 g Protein: 5.3 g

Simple Crepes

Crepes are a very thin pancake and are made in a similar manner. The biggest difference is that you have a thin batter that you roll around the pan to coat the entire surface. A true crepe pan is shallow and about 10 inches across. This recipe uses a smaller omelet pan, which works well and makes it easier to turn the crepe. There is a bit of a knack to doing it, so don't be discouraged if your first ones turn out broken or messy. (Pictured on page 136.)

1 Egg
1/3 cup Low Carb Flour
1/4 cup Heavy Cream
1/4 cup water
1 pinch Salt
1 teaspoon Oil

Use a blender or food processor to mix all ingredient together until smooth. Cover and refrigerate for at least one hour.

Heat a crepe pan or rounded 6 to 8 inch skillet over medium heat, then brush with oil. Pour 1/2 cup of the batter into the pan, then tilt it and roll the batter around to completely cover the pan's surface. Cook from three to four minutes, then gently ease a wide spatula under the crepe and turn it to cook the other side. Crepe should be a golden color.

Repeat to make other three crepes. Makes 4 crepes.

Nutrition Info:
Calories:104 Fat:9 g Net Carbs: 0.8g Protein: 4 g

You can use crepes with many different fillings. Add a little sugar substitute to the batter to make a sweeter crepe, then spread softened and sweetened cream cheese over it and top with sliced strawberries. Fold it over and put a few more strawberries and whipped cream on top. Delicious!

Cheese Taco Shells

As an alternative to low carb tortillas, these cheese taco shells are a fine option and easy to make. All you need to make them is a non-stick pan or griddle, a silicon spatula, and a foil-wrapped toilet paper or towel core roll for shaping the shell once it is cooked. (Pictured on page 136.)

For each taco shell:
1/2 cup Sharp Cheddar Cheese, Cheddar Jack Cheese
    or Provolone (2 slices)
1/2 teaspoon Golden Flax Meal (optional)
1/4 teaspoon Cayenne Pepper
Sprinkle of Garlic Powder
¼ teaspoon dried Cilantro

Skillet Method: In a small bowl, mix the ingredients together. Heat the non-stick skillet or griddle over medium high heat. Use your fingers to sprinkle the ingredients into the skillet making a 6" circle. Cook until the cheese is melted and bubbling, and just starting to crisp around the edges. Remove from heat. Use the spatula to carefully lift the cheese circle. Quickly, put the foil covered roll in the middle and fold the circle over it to form the shape. Slide the spatula under the bottom and place on a plate to cool until it is set. Remove the foil roll. The shell will hold its shape.

Microwave Method: Easiest way to make these. Lay a piece of parchment paper on a flat plate. Spread the cheese mixture to make a six inch circle. Microwave on high for 1 minute to 1 minute 20 seconds, depending on your microwave. The cheese should be melted and bubbly. Remove, let cool a few seconds until you can easily lift the cheese on one side. Place the foil covered roll in the middle and use the parchment paper to lift the shell over the roll. Let cool, then remove the roll.

Oven Method: If you want to make several at once, the oven method may work better. Preheat oven to 400 degrees (F). Line a cookie sheet with parchment paper. Mix 4 times as much cheese and seasonings. Spread cheese in four circles on the sheet. Bake for about 8 to 10 minutes until the cheese is melted and looks bubbly. Remove and use a spatula to carefully lift one side once the cheese is set. Roll around the foil wrapped roll. You will need to work quickly with these.

Repeat for each shell you wish to make.

Nutrition Info per shell -
  Sharp Cheddar:
    Calories: 228 Fat:18.6 g Net Carbs:2.6 g Protein: 12.4 g

  Cheddar Jack Cheese
    Calories: 174.6 Fat: 14.2 g Net Carbs: 2.1 g Protein: 14.0 g

  Provolone Cheese
    Calories: 148 Fat: 12.6 g Net Carbs: 0.6 g Protein: 10.4 g

Flax Meal Focaccia Bread

This is a small batch version that will make four squares of focaccia bread. Each square may be cut in half to make two slices for a sandwich or only use one half for an open-faced sandwich. (Pictured on page 136.)

1/2 cup ground Flax Meal
1/2 cup Almond Flour
1/2 tablespoon Baking Powder
1/2 teaspoon Salt
1/2 teaspoon Italian Seasoning
1/2 tablespoon Sugar Substitute
2 beaten Eggs
1 Egg White, okay to use packaged liquid
1/4 cup Water
3 tablespoons Olive Oil or Coconut Oil

Preheat Oven to 350 degrees (F.) Prepare an 8x8" square pan by cutting a piece of parchment paper to fit, then spray with cooking spray.

Mix your dry ingredients in a medium sized bowl. Mix the eggs, water and oil in a small bowl with a whisk. Make a well in the dry ingredients, then add the egg mixture and stir together until it's well mixed. You don't want any strings of egg white in your batter.

Spoon batter into the pan, putting an equal amount in all four corners, then use the back of a spoon to smooth it out to make an even layer.

Bake about 20 minutes until it springs back when you press the top. It should be lightly browned.

Cool and cut into 4" x 4" squares for sandwiches. Each square is thick enough to cut in half. Makes 4 sandwich rolls.

Nutrition Info per square
Calories: 219 Fat: 17.3g Net Carbs: 2.2 g Protein: 9.6 g

Special Ingredients

While I have tried to avoid using too many special ingredients in this cookbook, there are some that I have used and may be optional in the recipes. I am trying to keep the recipes as low carb as possible and this involves using ingredients that are manufactured with low carb dieters and diabetics in mind. In baking, the flours used are either nut flours or ones that are greatly reduced in wheat to create a low carb flour. While these don't taste exactly like the commercially produced flours, they do make a bread product that is very tasty and still good for you. In some cases, I actually prefer the taste of the low carb breads.

Flours

There are several manufacturers who create low carb baking mixes and flours. Among them are:

Tova Foods – makers of carbolose and CarbQuick Baking Mix

LC Foods – makers of many types of flours and mixes to help make low carb, gluten free baked goods, including cookies, cakes and bread. They also sell low carb jams and other products.

Dixie Carb Counters – makers of their own baking mix, many package mixes for breads, cheesecake, cookies and other meals.

New Hope Mills – makers of two fabulous muffin bread mixes and pancake mixes. I keep hoping they will expand their low carb line.

NOW Foods – makers of almond flour and coconut flour as well as other baking products.

Bob's Red Mill – a mill that you might find in your local grocery store. BRM produces almond flour, soy flour, hazelnut flour, a low carb baking mix, flax meal and other grains.

Ideal Foods – makes almond flour, flax meal and several other flours that are sold in grocery stores.

Not all low carb flours are created equal. Check the net carb (total carbohydrates minus fiber) count on the flours before using them. I generally use the lowest ones I can find, so if you use a baking mix that is 5 net carbs for 1/2 cup, then you'll be 2 carbs higher on the whole recipe than I am. As it is, the nutrition information may vary a little depending on how you measure, how large a particular vegetable may be and how you divide the dough up when baking.

Sugars

Sugar substitutes are controversial and are often in the news as not being all that good for you. I can only counter with the realization that sugar isn't that good for you either, especially when it packs the pounds on. You can completely give up sugar, but it's not easy to bake anything without some sweetener in it. Honey is not low carb and neither are any of the other syrups that are offered as a replacement.

There are quite a few brands of sweetener on the market. Generally, if the package is pink, it is a saccharin-based sweetener. If it is blue, then is aspartame-based. A yellow package is surcralose-based and if it is green, then it tends toward stevia.

More recently sugar alcohols have come into the market, but they aren't found as easily at the grocery store. They are not actually an alcohol, but a product produced from sugar. They are 0 calories and 0 carbs, but they don't agree with everyone's digestive system. Too much can cause stomach problems, so it's best to mix it with other sugar substitutes.

One of the things to keep in mind with any of the sugar substitutes, except the sugar alcohols, is that the actual sweetener is 0 carbs, but the medium used to carry the product—the powder in the package—has a little bit, less than 1 gram, of carbohydrate in it. It isn't a problem when you don't use it often, but if you are baking with it, a half cup of sugar substitute can add a few carbs to the count.

Other Baking Products

Some of the other powders and grains I use in my baking are low carb products that add texture and additional flavor to the finished goods. Among these:

Whey Protein Powder adds more protein, texture and flavor to bread products as well as making low carb shakes. It comes unflavored and in vanilla, chocolate and strawberry. It is not inexpensive, but I use only a tablespoon or two in baking.

Oat Fiber adds texture and maybe a bit of flavor, but it isn't noticeable. It also adds more fiber to the baked goods.

Egg White Powder adds more lift to the baked goods, but you can accomplish this by adding an egg white to the mix instead of the powder. When baking with coconut flour, extra egg whites are a must if you want it to rise at all. Baking powder and baking soda have no effect on coconut flour.

That said, I wish you all happy cooking and hope that this cookbook will open up some new possibilities for you. Please check out my blog [http://reneaverett.me/skinnygirl/] for more recipes and look for more cookbooks in the near future. I will be launching **Holiday Baking: Low Carb Recipe Magic** in November, 2015.

Conversion Tables

A few conversion tables to help non-Americans figure out the temperatures and measures. Amounts are approximate.

Oven Temperature Conversions

Fahrenheit	Celsius	Gas Mark
275° F	140° C	1 - cool
300° F	150° C	2
325° F	165° C	3
350° F	180° C	4 - moderate
375° F	190° C	5
400° F	200° C	6
425° F	220° C	7 – hot
450° F	230° C	9
475° F	240° C	10- very hot

Selected Food Equivalents & Yields

Butter	1 T.	14 grams	1 tablespoon	1/8 cup
	4 T.	56 grams	4 tablespoons	1/4 cup
	8 T. -1 stick	113 grams	8 tablespoons	1/2 cup
Chocolate	1 oz.	40 grams	4 tablespoons	1/4 cup
	6 oz. chips	160 grams	16 tablespoons	grated
				1 cup
Cocoa powder	1 Tablespoon	7.0 grams	1 tablespoon	0.25 oz
	4 Tablespoons	27.8 grams	1/4 cup	1 oz.
	16 Tablespoons	111.2 grams	1 cup	3.9 oz.
Half & Half Cream	1/2 milk & 1/2 cream	10.5 to 18% butterfat	1 tablespoon	0.5 fl. Oz
Light Cream		18 % butterfat	1 tablespoon	0.5 fl. Oz.
Light Whipping Cream		26-30% butterfat	1 tablespoon	0.5 fl. Oz.
Heavy Cream		36% or more butterfat	1 tablespoon	0.5 fl. Oz
Double Cream		42% butterfat	1 tablespoon	0.5 fl. oz

Measures for Pans and Dishes

7x11 baking dish	18x28 centimeter baking dish
9x13 inch baking dish	22x32.5 centimeter baking dish
8x8 inch baking dish	20x20 centimeter baking dish
9x5 inch loaf pan (8 cups capacity)	23x12 centimeter loaf pan (2 liter capacity)
10 inch tart or cake pan	25 centimeter tart or cake pan
9 inch cake pan	23 centimeter cake pan

ABOUT THE AUTHOR

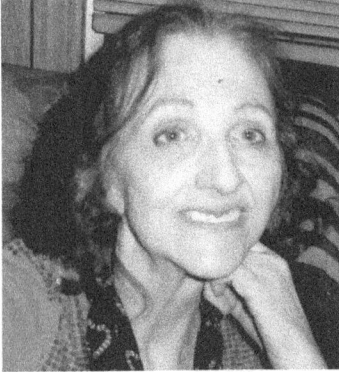

Rene Averett blogs regularly on her Skinny Girl Bistro site where she shares information about low carb foods, living a low carb lifestyle and many recipes. This is her first cookbook and it came about by the necessity of adapting recipes to her low carb lifestyle.

Rene hails from El Paso, Texas a good many years ago. She has lived in Los Angeles and Las Vegas and has made her home in Reno, Nevada since 1977. The latter part of her career centered on doing technical writing for a large gaming manufacturer and she enjoyed it right up until her retirement. She is now pursuing a career as an author and e-book publisher under Pynhavyn Press. She is a member of the Fiction Writers Group and the High Sierra Writers.

She loves the view of both the beautiful Sierra Nevada Mountains and the Virginia City Foothills from her house in South Reno that she shares with her long time companion, a dog, and four cats. She attempts a bit of gardening, loves to read and write fantasy, suspense romance and paranormal mystery novels.

Feedback is welcome. You can contact her via her website at: http://reneaverett.me/skinnygirl/ or at Rene@pynhavyn.com

You can also connect at her Facebook page, Skinny Girl Bistro at: https://www.facebook.com/sgbistro

www.ingramcontent.com/pod-product-compliance
Lightning Source LLC
Chambersburg PA
CBHW060443040426

42331CB00044B/2569